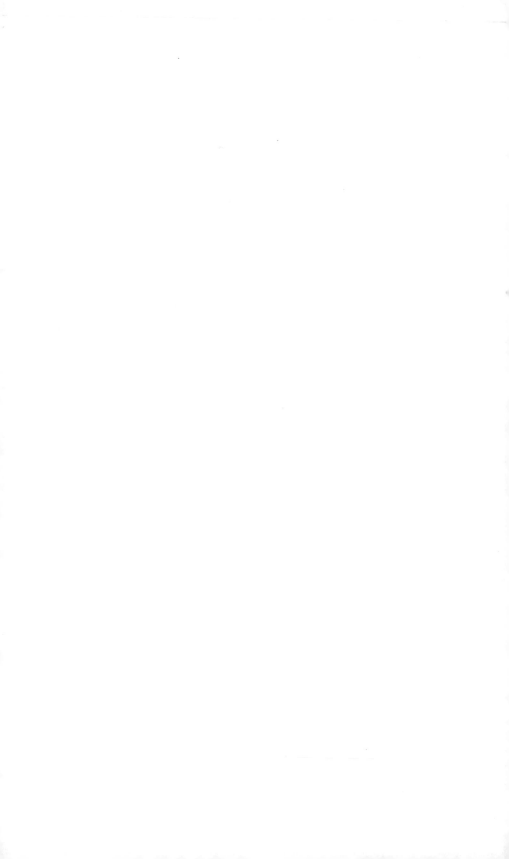

TOXICITY TESTING IN THE 21ST CENTURY
A VISION AND A STRATEGY

Committee on Toxicity Testing and Assessment of Environmental Agents

Board on Environmental Studies and Toxicology

Institute for Laboratory Animal Research

Division on Earth and Life Studies

NATIONAL RESEARCH COUNCIL
OF THE NATIONAL ACADEMIES

THE NATIONAL ACADEMIES PRESS
Washington, D.C.
www.nap.edu

THE NATIONAL ACADEMIES PRESS   500 Fifth Street, NW   Washington, DC 20001

NOTICE: The project that is the subject of this report was approved by the Governing Board of the National Research Council, whose members are drawn from the councils of the National Academy of Sciences, the National Academy of Engineering, and the Institute of Medicine. The members of the committee responsible for the report were chosen for their special competences and with regard for appropriate balance.

This project was supported by Contract 68-C-03-081 between the National Academy of Sciences and the U.S. Environmental Protection Agency. Any opinions, findings, conclusions, or recommendations expressed in this publication are those of the authors and do not necessarily reflect the view of the organizations or agencies that provided support for this project.

International Standard Book Number-13: 978-0-309-10992-5 (Book)
International Standard Book Number-10: 0-309-10992-2 (Book)
International Standard Book Number-13: 978-0-309-10993-2 (PDF)
International Standard Book Number-10: 0-309-10993-0 (PDF)
Library of Congress Control Number: 2007935052

Additional copies of this report are available from

The National Academies Press
500 Fifth Street, NW
Box 285
Washington, DC 20055

800-624-6242
202-334-3313 (in the Washington metropolitan area)
http://www.nap.edu

Copyright 2007 by the National Academy of Sciences. All rights reserved.

Printed in the United States of America.

THE NATIONAL ACADEMIES
Advisers to the Nation on Science, Engineering, and Medicine

The **National Academy of Sciences** is a private, nonprofit, self-perpetuating society of distinguished scholars engaged in scientific and engineering research, dedicated to the furtherance of science and technology and to their use for the general welfare. Upon the authority of the charter granted to it by the Congress in 1863, the Academy has a mandate that requires it to advise the federal government on scientific and technical matters. Dr. Ralph J. Cicerone is president of the National Academy of Sciences.

The **National Academy of Engineering** was established in 1964, under the charter of the National Academy of Sciences, as a parallel organization of outstanding engineers. It is autonomous in its administration and in the selection of its members, sharing with the National Academy of Sciences the responsibility for advising the federal government. The National Academy of Engineering also sponsors engineering programs aimed at meeting national needs, encourages education and research, and recognizes the superior achievements of engineers. Dr. Charles M. Vest is president of the National Academy of Engineering.

The **Institute of Medicine** was established in 1970 by the National Academy of Sciences to secure the services of eminent members of appropriate professions in the examination of policy matters pertaining to the health of the public. The Institute acts under the responsibility given to the National Academy of Sciences by its congressional charter to be an adviser to the federal government and, upon its own initiative, to identify issues of medical care, research, and education. Dr. Harvey V. Fineberg is president of the Institute of Medicine.

The **National Research Council** was organized by the National Academy of Sciences in 1916 to associate the broad community of science and technology with the Academy's purposes of furthering knowledge and advising the federal government. Functioning in accordance with general policies determined by the Academy, the Council has become the principal operating agency of both the National Academy of Sciences and the National Academy of Engineering in providing services to the government, the public, and the scientific and engineering communities. The Council is administered jointly by both Academies and the Institute of Medicine. Dr. Ralph J. Cicerone and Dr. Charles M. Vest are chair and vice chair, respectively, of the National Research Council.

www.national-academies.org

COMMITTEE ON TOXICITY TESTING AND ASSESSMENT OF ENVIRONMENTAL AGENTS

Members

DANIEL KREWSKI (*Chair*), University of Ottawa, ON, Canada
DANIEL ACOSTA, JR., University of Cincinnati, OH
MELVIN ANDERSEN, The Hamner Institutes for Health Sciences, Research Triangle Park, NC
HENRY ANDERSON, Wisconsin Division of Public Health, Madison
JOHN BAILAR III, University of Chicago, IL
KIM BOEKELHEIDE, Brown University, Providence, RI
ROBERT BRENT, Thomas Jefferson University, Wilmington, DE
GAIL CHARNLEY, HealthRisk Strategies, Washington, DC
VIVIAN CHEUNG, University of Pennsylvania, Philadelphia
SIDNEY GREEN, Howard University, Washington, DC
KARL KELSEY, Harvard University, Boston, MA
NANCY KERKVLIET, Oregon State University, Corvallis
ABBY LI, Exponent, Inc., San Francisco, CA
LAWRENCE MCCRAY, Massachusetts Institute of Technology, Cambridge
OTTO MEYER, The National Food Institute, Technical University of Denmark, Søborg, Denmark
D. REID PATTERSON, Reid Patterson Consulting, Inc., Elkhorn, WI
WILLIAM PENNIE, Pfizer, Inc., Groton, CT
ROBERT SCALA, Exxon Biomedical Sciences (Ret.), Tucson, AZ
GINA SOLOMON, Natural Resources Defense Council, San Francisco, CA
MARTIN STEPHENS, The Humane Society of the United States, Washington, DC
JAMES YAGER, JR., Johns Hopkins University, Baltimore, MD
LAUREN ZEISE, California Environmental Protection Agency, Oakland

Staff

ELLEN MANTUS, Project Director
JENNIFER OBERNIER, Program Officer
RUTH CROSSGROVE, Senior Editor
NORMAN GROSSBLATT, Senior Editor
MIRSADA KARALIC-LONCAREVIC, Manager, Technical Information Center
JORDAN CRAGO, Senior Project Assistant

Sponsor

U.S. ENVIRONMENTAL PROTECTION AGENCY

BOARD ON ENVIRONMENTAL STUDIES AND TOXICOLOGY

Members

JONATHAN M. SAMET (*Chair*), Johns Hopkins University, Baltimore, MD
RAMÓN ALVAREZ, Environmental Defense, Austin, TX
JOHN M. BALBUS, Environmental Defense, Washington, DC
DALLAS BURTRAW, Resources for the Future, Washington, DC
JAMES S. BUS, Dow Chemical Company, Midland, MI
COSTEL D. DENSON, University of Delaware, Newark
E. DONALD ELLIOTT, Willkie Farr & Gallagher LLP, Washington, DC
MARY R. ENGLISH, University of Tennessee, Knoxville
RUTH DEFRIES, University of Maryland, College Park
J. PAUL GILMAN, Oak Ridge Center for Advanced Studies, Oak Ridge, TN
SHERRI W. GOODMAN, Center for Naval Analyses, Alexandria, VA
JUDITH A. GRAHAM, American Chemistry Council, Arlington, VA
WILLIAM P. HORN, Birch, Horton, Bittner and Cherot, Washington, DC
WILLIAM M. LEWIS, JR., University of Colorado, Boulder
JUDITH L. MEYER, University of Georgia, Athens
DENNIS D. MURPHY, University of Nevada, Reno
PATRICK Y. O'BRIEN, ChevronTexaco Energy Technology Company, Richmond, CA
DOROTHY E. PATTON (retired), Chicago, IL
DANNY D. REIBLE, University of Texas, Austin
JOSEPH V. RODRICKS, ENVIRON International Corporation, Arlington, VA
ARMISTEAD G. RUSSELL, Georgia Institute of Technology, Atlanta
ROBERT F. SAWYER, University of California, Berkeley
KIMBERLY M. THOMPSON, Massachusetts Institute of Technology, Cambridge
MONICA G. TURNER, University of Wisconsin, Madison
MARK J. UTELL, University of Rochester Medical Center, Rochester, NY
CHRIS G. WHIPPLE, ENVIRON International Corporation, Emeryville, CA
LAUREN ZEISE, California Environmental Protection Agency, Oakland

Senior Staff

JAMES J. REISA, Director
DAVID J. POLICANSKY, Scholar
RAYMOND A. WASSEL, Senior Program Officer for Environmental Sciences and Engineering
KULBIR BAKSHI, Senior Program Officer for Toxicology
EILEEN N. ABT, Senior Program Officer for Risk Analysis
KARL E. GUSTAVSON, Senior Program Officer
K. JOHN HOLMES, Senior Program Officer
ELLEN K. MANTUS, Senior Program Officer
SUSAN N.J. MARTEL, Senior Program Officer
STEVEN K. GIBB, Program Officer for Strategic Communications
RUTH E. CROSSGROVE, Senior Editor

vi

INSTITUTE FOR LABORATORY ANIMAL RESEARCH COUNCIL

Members

STEPHEN W. BARTHOLD *(Chair)*, University of California, Davis
KATHRYN A. BAYNE, Association for Assessment and Accreditation of Laboratory Animal Care International, Waikoloa, HI
MYRTLE A. DAVIS, Lilly Research Laboratories, Greenfield, IN
JEFFREY I. EVERITT, GlaxoSmithKline Research and Development, Research Triangle Park, NC
JAMES G. FOX, Massachusetts Institute of Technology, Cambridge
NELSON L. GARNETT, (formerly) Johns Hopkins University, Baltimore, MD
ESTELLE B. GAUDA, Johns Hopkins University, Baltimore, MD
COENRAAD F.M. HENDRIKSEN, Netherlands Vaccine Institute, Bilthoven
JON H. KAAS, Vanderbilt University, Nashville, TN
JOSEPH W. KEMNITZ, University of Wisconsin, Madison
JUDY A. MCARTHUR CLARK, (formerly) Pfizer Global R&D, Groton, CT
LETICIA V. MEDINA, Abbott Laboratories, Abbott Park, IL
BERNARD E. ROLLIN, Colorado State University, Fort Collins
ABIGAIL L. SMITH, University of Pennsylvania, Philadelphia
STEPHEN A. SMITH, Virginia Polytechnic Institute and State University, Blacksburg

Staff

JOANNE ZURLO, Director
LIDA ANESTIDOU, Program Officer
KATHLEEN BEIL, Administrative Coordinator
RHONDA HAYCRAFT, Senior Project Assistant
SUSAN VAUPEL, Managing Editor, *ILAR Journal*

OTHER REPORTS OF THE
BOARD ON ENVIRONMENTAL STUDIES AND TOXICOLOGY

Models in Environmental Regulatory Decision Making (2007)
Sediment Dredging at Superfund Megasites: Assessing the Effectiveness (2007)
Environmental Impacts of Wind-Energy Projects (2007)
Scientific Review of the Proposed Risk Assessment Bulletin from the Office of Management and Budget (2007)
Assessing the Human Health Risks of Trichloroethylene: Key Scientific Issues (2006)
New Source Review for Stationary Sources of Air Pollution (2006)
Human Biomonitoring for Environmental Chemicals (2006)
Health Risks from Dioxin and Related Compounds: Evaluation of the EPA Reassessment (2006)
Fluoride in Drinking Water: A Scientific Review of EPA's Standards (2006)
State and Federal Standards for Mobile-Source Emissions (2006)
Superfund and Mining Megasites—Lessons from the Coeur d'Alene River Basin (2005)
Health Implications of Perchlorate Ingestion (2005)
Air Quality Management in the United States (2004)
Endangered and Threatened Species of the Platte River (2004)
Atlantic Salmon in Maine (2004)
Endangered and Threatened Fishes in the Klamath River Basin (2004)
Cumulative Environmental Effects of Alaska North Slope Oil and Gas Development (2003)
Estimating the Public Health Benefits of Proposed Air Pollution Regulations (2002)
Biosolids Applied to Land: Advancing Standards and Practices (2002)
The Airliner Cabin Environment and Health of Passengers and Crew (2002)
Arsenic in Drinking Water: 2001 Update (2001)
Evaluating Vehicle Emissions Inspection and Maintenance Programs (2001)
Compensating for Wetland Losses Under the Clean Water Act (2001)
A Risk-Management Strategy for PCB-Contaminated Sediments (2001)
Acute Exposure Guideline Levels for Selected Airborne Chemicals (five volumes, 2000-2007)
Toxicological Effects of Methylmercury (2000)
Strengthening Science at the U.S. Environmental Protection Agency (2000)
Scientific Frontiers in Developmental Toxicology and Risk Assessment (2000)
Ecological Indicators for the Nation (2000)
Waste Incineration and Public Health (2000)
Hormonally Active Agents in the Environment (1999)
Research Priorities for Airborne Particulate Matter (four volumes, 1998-2004)
The National Research Council's Committee on Toxicology: The First 50 Years (1997)
Carcinogens and Anticarcinogens in the Human Diet (1996)
Upstream: Salmon and Society in the Pacific Northwest (1996)
Science and the Endangered Species Act (1995)
Wetlands: Characteristics and Boundaries (1995)
Biologic Markers (five volumes, 1989-1995)
Review of EPA's Environmental Monitoring and Assessment Program (three volumes, 1994-1995)
Science and Judgment in Risk Assessment (1994)

Pesticides in the Diets of Infants and Children (1993)
Dolphins and the Tuna Industry (1992)
Science and the National Parks (1992)
Human Exposure Assessment for Airborne Pollutants (1991)
Rethinking the Ozone Problem in Urban and Regional Air Pollution (1991)
Decline of the Sea Turtles (1990)

Copies of these reports may be ordered from the National Academies Press
(800) 624-6242 or (202) 334-3313
www.nap.edu

INSTITUTE FOR LABORATORY ANIMAL RESEARCH PUBLICATIONS

Science, Medicine, and Animals: A Circle of Discovery (2004)
The Development of Science-Based Guidelines for Laboratory Animal Care: Proceedings of the November 2003 International Workshop (2004)
National Need and Priorities for Veterinarians in Biomedical Research (2004)
Occupational Health and Safety in the Care and Use of Nonhuman Primates (2003)
International Perspectives—The Future of Nonhuman Primate Resources: Proceedings of the Workshop Held April 17-19, 2002 (2003)
Guidelines for the Care and Use of Mammals in Neuroscience and Behavioral Research (2003)
Principles and Guidelines for the Use of Animals in Precollege Education (2001)
Strategies That Influence Cost Containment in Animal Research (2000)
Definition of Pain and Distress and Reporting Requirements for Laboratory Animals: Proceedings of the Workshop Held June 22, 2000 (2000)
Monoclonal Antibody Production (1999)
Microbial and Phenotypic Definition of Rats and Mice: Proceedings of the 1999 US/Japan Conference (1999)
The Psychological Well-Being of Nonhuman Primates (1998)
Microbial Status and Genetic Evaluation of Mice and Rats: Proceedings of the 1998 US/Japan Conference (1998)
Biomedical Models and Resources: Current Needs and Future Opportunities (1998)
Approaches to Cost Recovery for Animal Research: Implications for Science, Animals, Research Competitiveness, and Regulatory Compliance (1998)
Occupational Health and Safety in the Care and Use of Research Animals (1997)
Chimpanzees in Research: Strategies for Their Ethical Care, Management, and Use (1997)
Guide for the Care and Use of Laboratory Animals, 7th ed. (1996)
Nutrient Requirements of Laboratory Animals, 4th ed. (1995)
Laboratory Animal Management: Dogs (1994)
Recognition and Alleviation of Pain and Distress in Laboratory Animals (1992)
Infectious Diseases of Mice and Rats (1991)
Companion Guide to Infectious Diseases of Mice and Rats (1991)
Laboratory Animal Management: Rodents (1990)
Immunodeficient Rodents: A Guide to Their Immunobiology, Husbandry, and Use (1989)
Use of Laboratory Animals in Biomedical and Behavioral Research (1988)

Copies of these reports may be ordered from the National Academies Press
(800) 624-6242 or (202) 334-3313
www.nap.edu

Preface

Over the past few decades, several toxicity-testing strategies have emerged for evaluating the hazards or risks associated with exposure to drugs, food additives, pesticides, and industrial and other chemicals. New testing technologies, methods, and approaches also have emerged in recent years. The U.S. Environmental Protection Agency (EPA) recognized the need to conduct a comprehensive review of toxicity-testing methods and strategies and requested that the National Research Council (NRC) conduct such a review and propose a long-range vision and strategy for toxicity testing.

In its 2006 interim report, the NRC Committee on Toxicity Testing and Assessment of Environmental Agents reviewed current toxicity-testing methods and strategies and selected aspects of several reports by EPA and others that described initiatives or proposals to improve current methods or strategies. The committee now presents its long-range vision and strategic plan to advance toxicity testing and considers its vision within the current regulatory framework. Although the committee was not charged to review government programs related to toxicity testing, some federal programs that are relevant to the subject of this report may be of interest to readers. For example, EPA has established a National Center for Computational Toxicology (http://www.epa.gov/comptox/index.html) that is developing new software and methods for predictive toxicology. The National Institute of Environmental Health Sciences, through the National Toxicology Program's Roadmap for the Future (http://ntp.niehs.nih.gov/files/NTPrdmp.pdf), has initiated a partnership with the Chemical Genomics Center of the National Institutes of Health to develop and carry out high- and medium-throughput screening assays to test more chemicals in less time and at less cost.

This report has been reviewed in draft form by persons chosen for their diverse perspectives and technical expertise in accordance with procedures approved by the NRC's Report Review Committee. The purposes of this independent review are to provide candid and critical comments that will assist the institution in making its published report as sound as possible and to ensure that the report meets institutional standards of objectivity, evidence, and responsiveness to the study charge. The review comments and draft manuscript remain confidential to protect the integrity of the deliberative process. We wish to thank the following for their review of this report: Cynthia Afshari (Amgen, Inc.), Frederic Bois (INERIS), James Bus (Dow Chemical), Vincent James Cogliano (International Agency for Research on Cancer), David Dorman (The Hamner Institutes for Health Sciences), Alan Goldberg (Johns Hopkins University), Carole Kimmel (consultant), Gilbert Omenn (University of Michigan), Lorenz Rhomberg (Gradient Corporation), Joseph Rodricks (ENVIRON), Leslie Stayner (University of Illinois), and Helmut Zarbl (Fred Hutchinson Cancer Research Center).

Although the reviewers listed above have provided many constructive comments and suggestions, they were not asked to endorse the conclusions or recommendations, nor did they see the final draft of the report before its release. The review of this report was overseen by the review coordinator, Rogene Henderson (Lovelace Respiratory Research Institute), and the review monitor, Donald Mattison (National Institutes of Health). Appointed by the NRC, they were responsible for making certain that an independent examination of this report was carried out in accordance with institutional procedures and that all review comments were carefully considered. Responsibility for the final content of this report rests entirely with the committee and the institution.

The committee gratefully acknowledges the following for making presentations to the committee: Thomas Hartung (ECVAM), William Greenlee (The Hamner Institutes for Health Sciences), Carl Barrett (Novartis Institute for Bio-Medical Development), Robert Chapin (Pfizer, Inc.), Michael Festing (private consultant), William Stokes (National Institute of Environmental Health Sciences), Edward Calabrese (University of Massachusetts-Amherst), John Doull (University of Kansas Medical Center), Bette Meek (Health Canada), Michael Firestone (EPA), Clifford Gabriel (EPA), Lee Hoffman (EPA), Jim Jones (EPA), Deidre Murphy (EPA), Rita Schoeny (EPA), and Charles Auer (EPA). The committee especially thanks Dorothy Patton (retired from EPA) for her contributions to the report and consultation on toxicity testing in regulatory contexts.

The committee is also grateful for the assistance of the NRC staff in preparing this report. Staff members who contributed to the effort are Ellen Mantus, project director; Joanne Zurlo, director of the Institute for Laboratory Animal Research; James Reisa, director of the Board on Environmental Studies and Toxicology; Jennifer Obernier, program officer; Ruth Crossgrove, senior editor; Norman Grossblatt, senior editor; Mirsada Karalic-Loncarevic, manager of the Technical Information Center; Jordan Crago, senior project assistant; and Radiah Rose, senior editorial assistant.

I would especially like to thank all the members of the committee for their efforts throughout the development of this report.

Daniel Krewski, *Chair*
Committee on Toxicity Testing
and Assessment of Environmental Agents

Contents

Contents

Contents

TOXICITY TESTING IN THE 21ST CENTURY

A VISION AND A STRATEGY

Summary

Change often involves a pivotal event that builds on previous history and opens the door to a new era. Pivotal events in science include the discovery of penicillin, the elucidation of the DNA double helix, and the development of computers. All were marked by inauspicious beginnings followed by unheralded advances over a period of years but ultimately resulted in a pharmacopoeia of life-saving drugs, a map of the human genome, and a personal computer on almost every desk in today's workplace.

Toxicity testing is approaching such a scientific pivot point. It is poised to take advantage of the revolutions in biology and biotechnology. Advances in toxicogenomics, bioinformatics, systems biology, epigenetics, and computational toxicology could transform toxicity testing from a system based on whole-animal testing to one founded primarily on in vitro methods that evaluate changes in biologic processes using cells, cell lines, or cellular components, preferably of human origin. Anticipating the impact of recent scientific advances, the U.S. Environmental Protection Agency (EPA) asked the National Research Council (NRC) to develop a long-range vision for toxicity testing and a strategic plan for implementing the vision.

This report of the NRC Committee on Toxicity Testing and Assessment of Environmental Agents, prepared in response to EPA's request, envisions a major campaign in the scientific community to advance the science of toxicity testing and put it on a forward-looking footing. The potential benefits are clear. Fresh thinking and the use of emerging methods for understanding how environmental agents affect human health will promote beneficial changes in testing of these agents and in the use of data for decision-making. The envisioned change is expected to generate more robust data on the potential risks to humans posed by exposure to environmental agents and to expand capabilities to test chemicals more efficiently. A stronger scientific foundation offers the prospect of improved risk-based regulatory decisions and possibly greater public confidence in and acceptance of the decisions.

With those goals in mind, the committee presents in this report a vision for mobilizing the scientific community and marshalling scientific resources to initiate and sustain new approaches, some available and others yet to be developed, to toxicity testing. This report speaks to scientists in all sectors—government, public interest, industry, university, and consulting laboratories—who design and conduct toxicity tests and who use test results to evaluate risks to human health. The report also seeks to inform and engage decision-makers and other leaders who shape the nature and scope of government regulations and who establish budgetary priorities that will determine progress in advancing toxicity testing in the future. The full impact of the committee's wide-ranging recommendations can be achieved only if both scientists and nonscientists work to advance the objectives set forth in the vision.

THE VISION

The current approach to toxicity testing relies primarily on a complex array of studies that evaluate observable outcomes in whole animals, such as clinical signs or pathologic changes, that are indicative of a disease state. Partly because that strategy is so time-consuming and resource-intensive, it has had difficulty in meeting many challenges encountered today, such as evaluating various life stages, numerous health outcomes, and large numbers of untested chemicals. The committee debated several options for improving the current system but concluded that a transformative paradigm shift is needed to achieve the design criteria set out in the committee's interim report: (1) to provide broad coverage of chemicals, chemical mixtures, outcomes, and life stages, (2) to reduce the cost and time of testing, (3) to use fewer animals and cause minimal suffering in the animals used, and (4) to develop a more robust scientific basis for assessing health effects of environmental agents.[1]

The committee considered recent scientific advances in defining a new approach to toxicity testing. Substantial progress is being made in the elucidation of cellular-response networks— interconnected pathways composed of complex biochemical interactions of genes, proteins, and small molecules that maintain normal cellular function, control communication between cells, and allow cells to adapt to changes in their environment. For example, one familiar cellular-response network is signaling by estrogens in which initial exposure results in enhanced cell proliferation and tissue growth in specific tissues. Bioscience is enhancing our knowledge of cellular-response networks and allowing scientists to begin to uncover how environmental agents perturb pathways in ways that lead to toxicity. Cellular response pathways that, when sufficiently perturbed, are expected to result

---

[1]For a further discussion of the options considered by the committee, see Chapter 2, "Options for a New Toxicity-Testing Paradigm."

in adverse health effects are termed *toxicity pathways*. The commit-tee envisions a new toxicity-testing system that evaluates biologi-cally significant perturbations in key toxicity pathways by using new methods in computational biology and a comprehensive array of in vitro tests based on human biology.

COMPONENTS OF THE VISION

Figure S-1 illustrates the major components of the commit-tee's vision: chemical characterization, toxicity testing, and dose-response and extrapolation modeling. The components of the vi-sion, which are described in the sections that follow, are distinct but interrelated modules involving specific sets of technologies and scientific capabilities. Some chemical evaluations may pro-ceed in a stepwise manner—from chemical characterization to tox-icity testing to dose-response and extrapolation modeling—but such a sequential evaluation need not always be followed in prac-tice. A critical feature of the new vision is consideration of the risk context (the decision-making context that creates the need for tox-icity-testing information) at each step and the ability to exit the strategy at any point when sufficient data have been generated for decision-making. The vision emphasizes the generation and use of population-based and human exposure data where possible for interpreting test results and encourages the collection of such data on important chemicals with biomonitoring, surveillance, and epidemiologic studies. Population-based and human exposure data, along with the risk context, will play a role in both guiding and using the toxicity information that is produced. Finally, the vision anticipates the development of a formal process to phase in and phase out test methods as scientific understanding of toxicity-testing methods expands. That process addresses the need for effi-cient testing of all chemicals in a timely, cost-effective fashion.

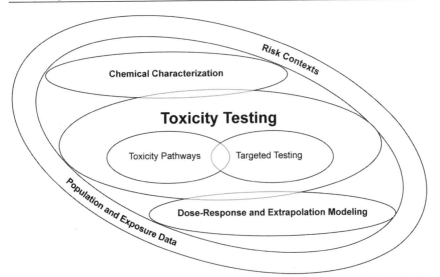

FIGURE S-1 The committee's vision for toxicity testing is a process that includes chemical characterization, toxicity testing, and dose-response and extrapolation modeling. At each step, population-based and human exposure data are considered, as is the question of what data are needed for decision-making.

Chemical Characterization

Chemical characterization is meant to provide insights to key questions, including a compound's stability in the environment, the potential for human exposure, the likely routes of exposure, the potential for bioaccumulation, possible routes of metabolism, and the likely toxicity of the compound and possible metabolites based on chemical structure or physical or chemical characteristics. Thus, data would be collected on physical and chemical properties, use, possible environmental concentrations, metabolites and breakdown products, initial molecular interactions of compounds and metabolites with cellular components, and possible toxic properties. A variety of computational methods might be used to predict those properties and characteristics. After chemical characterization, decisions might be made about what further testing is required or whether it is needed at all. In most cases, chemical characterization alone is not expected to be sufficient to reach decisions about the toxicity of an environmental agent.

Toxicity Testing

In the vision proposed (see Figure S-1), toxicity testing has two components: toxicity-pathway assays and targeted testing. The committee expects that when the vision is achieved, predictive, pathway-based assays will serve as the central component of a broad toxicity-testing strategy for assessing the biologic activity of new and existing compounds. Targeted testing will serve to complement the assays and support evaluation.

Toxicity Pathways

Figure S-2 illustrates the activation of a toxicity pathway. The initial perturbations of cell-signaling motifs, genetic circuits, and cellular-response networks are obligatory changes resulting from chemical exposure that might eventually result in disease. The consequences of a biologic perturbation depend on its magnitude, which is related to the dose, the timing and duration of the perturbation, and the susceptibility of the host. Accordingly, at low doses, many biologic systems may function normally within their homeostatic limits. At somewhat higher doses, clear biologic responses occur. They may be successfully handled by adaptation, although some susceptible people may respond. More intense or persistent perturbations may overwhelm the capacity of the system to adapt and lead to tissue injury and possible adverse health effects.

The committee's vision capitalizes on the identification and use of toxicity pathways as the basis of new approaches to toxicity

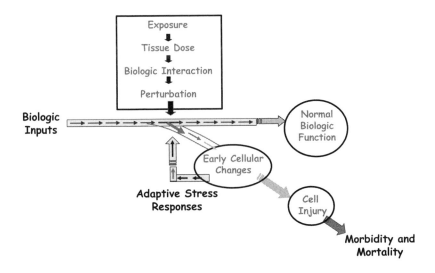

FIGURE S-2 Biologic responses viewed as results of an intersection of exposure and biologic function. The intersection results in perturbation of biologic pathways. When perturbations are sufficiently large or when the host is unable to adapt because of underlying nutritional, genetic, disease, or life-stage status, biologic function is compromised, and this leads to toxicity and disease. Source: Adapted from Andersen, M.E., J.E. Dennison, R.S. Thomas, and R.B. Conolly. 2005. New directions in incidence-dose modeling. Trends Biotechnol. 23(3):122-127. Reprinted with permission; copyright 2005, *Trends in Biotechnology*.

testing and dose-response modeling. Accordingly, the vision emphasizes the development of suites of predictive, high-throughput assays[2] that use cells or cell lines, preferably of human origin, to evaluate relevant perturbations in key toxicity pathways. Those assays may measure relatively simple processes, such as binding of environmental agents with cellular proteins and changes in gene expression caused by that binding, or they may measure

---

[2]High-throughput assays are efficiently designed experiments that can be automated and rapidly performed to measure the effect of substances on a biologic process of interest. These assays can evaluate hundreds to many thousands of chemicals over a wide concentration range to identify chemical actions on gene, pathway, and cell function.

more integrated responses, such as cell division and cell differentiation. Although the majority of toxicity tests in the vision are expected to use high-throughput methods, other tests could include medium-throughput assays of more integrated cellular responses, such as cytotoxicity, cell proliferation, and apoptosis. Over time, the need for traditional animal testing should be greatly reduced and possibly even eliminated.

Targeted Testing

Targeted testing would be used to complement toxicity-pathway tests and to ensure adequate evaluation. It would be used (1) to clarify substantial uncertainties in the interpretation of toxicity-pathway data; (2) to understand effects of representative prototype compounds from classes of materials, such as nanoparticles, that may activate toxicity pathways not included in a standard suite of assays; (3) to refine a risk estimate when the targeted testing can reduce uncertainty, and a more refined estimate is needed for decision-making; (4) to investigate the production of possibly toxic metabolites; and (5) to fill gaps in the toxicity-pathway testing strategy to ensure that critical toxicity pathways and end points are adequately covered. One of the challenges of developing an in vitro test system to evaluate toxicity is the current inability of cell assays to mirror metabolism in the integrated whole animal. For the foreseeable future, any in vitro strategy will need to include a provision to assess likely metabolites through whole-animal testing.

Targeted testing might be conducted in vivo or in vitro, depending on the toxicity tests available. Although targeted tests could be based on existing toxicity-test systems, they will probably differ from traditional tests in the future. They could use transgenic species, isogenic strains, new animal models, or other novel test systems and could include a toxicogenomic evaluation of tissue responses over wide dose ranges. Whatever system is used, testing protocols would maximize the amount of information gained from whole-animal toxicity testing.

Dose-Response and Extrapolation Modeling

In the vision proposed (see Figure S-1), dose-response models would be developed for environmental agents primarily on the basis of data from mechanistic, in vitro assays as described in the toxicity-testing component. The dose-response models would describe the relationship between concentration in the test medium and degree of in vitro response. In some risk contexts, a dose-response model based on in vitro results might provide adequate data to support a risk-management decision. An example could involve compounds for which host-susceptibility factors in humans are well understood and human biomonitoring provides good information about tissue or blood concentrations of the compound and other related exposures that affect the toxicity pathway in a human population.

Extrapolation modeling estimates the environmental exposures or human intakes that would lead to human tissue concentrations similar to those associated with perturbations of toxicity pathways in vitro and would account for host susceptibility factors. In the vision proposed, extrapolation modeling has three primary components. First, a toxicity-pathway model would provide a quantitative, mechanistic understanding of the dose-response relationship for the perturbations of the pathways by environmental agents. Second, physiologically based pharmacokinetic modeling would then be used to predict human exposures that lead to tissue concentrations that could be compared with the concentrations that caused perturbations in vitro. Third, human data would provide information on background chemical exposures and disease processes that would affect the same toxicity pathway and provide a basis for addressing host susceptibility quantitatively.

Population-Based and Human Exposure Data

Population-based and human exposure data are important components of the committee's toxicity-testing strategy (see Figure S-1). Those data can help to inform each component of the vision and ensure the integrity of the overall testing strategy. The shift toward the collection of more mechanistic data on fundamental biologic perturbations in human cells will require greater use of biomonitoring and human-surveillance studies for data interpretation. Moreover, the interaction between population-based studies and toxicity tests will improve the design of each study type for answering questions about the importance of molecular, cellular, and genetic factors that influence individual and population-level health risks. Because the vision emphasizes studies conducted in human cells that indicate how environmental agents can affect human biologic responses, the studies will suggest biomarkers (indicators of human exposure, effect, or susceptibility) that can be monitored and studied in human populations.

As toxicity testing shifts to cell-based studies, human exposure data from biomonitoring studies (such as those recommended in the NRC report *Human Biomonitoring for Environmental Chemicals*[3]) may prove pivotal. Such data can be used to select doses for toxicity testing that can provide information on biologic effects at environmentally relevant exposures. More important, comparison of concentrations that activate toxicity pathways with concentrations of agents in blood, urine, or other tissues from human populations will help to identify potentially important expo-

---

[3]NRC (National Research Council). 2006. *Human Biomonitoring for Environmental Chemicals*. Washington, DC: The National Academies Press.

sures to ensure an adequate margin of safety in setting human exposure guidelines.

Risk Context

Toxicity testing is useful ultimately only if it can be used to facilitate more informed and efficient responses to the public-health concerns of regulators, industry, and the public. Common scenarios, defined by the committee as "risk contexts," for which toxicity testing is used to make decisions include evaluation of potential environmental agents, existing environmental agents, sites of environmental contamination, environmental contributors to a human disease, and the relative risk of different environmental agents. Some risk contexts require rapid screening of tens of thousands of environmental agents; some require highly refined dose-response data, extending down to environmentally relevant exposure concentrations; and some require the ability to test chemical mixtures or to use assays focused on specific mechanisms. Some risk contexts might require the use of population-based approaches, including population health surveillance and biomonitoring. With its emphasis on high-throughput assays that use human cells, cell lines, and components to evaluate biologically significant perturbations in key toxicity pathways, the vision presented here will assist the decision-making process in each risk context.

IMPLEMENTATION OF THE VISION

Implementation of the vision will require (1) the availability of suites of in vitro tests—preferably based on human cells, cell lines, or components—that are sufficiently comprehensive to evaluate activity in toxicity pathways associated with the broad array of possible toxic responses; (2) the availability of targeted tests to complement the in vitro tests and ensure an adequate toxicity database for risk-management decision-making; (3) computational models of toxicity pathways to support application of in vitro test results to predict exposures in the general population that could potentially lead to adverse changes; (4) infrastructure changes to support the basic and applied research needed to develop the tests and the pathway models; (5) validation of tests and test strategies for incorporation into chemical-assessment guidelines that will provide direction in interpreting and drawing conclusions from the new assay results; and (6) evidence justifying that the results of tests based on perturbations in toxicity pathways are adequately predictive of adverse health outcomes to be used in decision-making.

A substantial and focused research effort will be needed to meet those requirements. The research will need to develop both new scientific knowledge and new toxicity-testing methods. Key questions that need to be addressed regarding knowledge and method development are highlighted in Box S-1.

The research and development needed to implement the vision would progress in phases whose timelines would overlap. Phase I would focus on elucidating toxicity pathways; developing a data-storage, -access, and -management system; developing standard protocols for research methods and reporting; and planning a strategy for human surveillance and biomonitoring to support the toxicity-pathway testing approach. Phase II would involve development and validation of toxicity-pathway assays and identification of markers of exposure, effect, and susceptibility for use in surveillance and biomonitoring of human populations. Phase III would evaluate assays by running them in parallel with traditional toxicity tests, on chemicals with large datasets, and on chemicals that would not otherwise be tested as a screening process. Parallel testing will allow identification of toxicities that might

---

BOX S-1 Key Questions to Address in Implementation

Knowledge Development

Toxicity-Pathway Identification—What are the key pathways whose perturbations result in toxicity?

Multiple Pathways—What alteration in response can be expected from simultaneous perturbations of multiple toxicity pathways?

Adversity—What adverse effects are linked to specific toxicity-pathway perturbations? What patterns and magnitudes of perturbations are predictive of adverse health outcomes?

Life Stages—How can the perturbations of toxicity pathways associated with developmental timing or aging be best captured to enable the advancement of high-throughput assays?

Effects of Exposure Duration—How are biologic responses affected by exposures of different duration?

Low-Dose Response—What is the effect on a toxicity pathway of adding small amounts of toxicants in light of pre-existing endogenous and exogenous human exposures?

Human Variability—How do people differ in their expression of toxicity-pathway constituents and in their predisposition to disease and impairment?

Method Development

Methods to Predict Metabolism—How can adequate testing for metabolites in the high-throughput assays be ensured?

Chemical-Characterization Tools—What computational tools can best predict chemical properties, metabolites, xenobiotic-cellular and molecular interactions, and biologic activity?

Assays to Uncover Cell Circuitry—What methods will best facilitate the discovery of the circuitry associated with toxicity pathways?

Assays for Large-Scale Application—Which assays best capture the elucidated pathways and best reflect in vivo conditions? What designs will ensure adequate testing of volatile compounds?

(Continued on next page)

BOX S-1 Continued

Suite of Assays—What mix of pathway-based high- and medium-throughput assays and targeted tests will provide adequate coverage? What targeted tests should be developed to complement the toxicity-pathway assays? What are the appropriate positive and negative controls that should be used to validate the assay suite?

Human-Surveillance Strategy—What surveillance is needed to interpret the results of pathway tests in light of variable human susceptibility and background exposures?

Mathematical Models for Data Interpretation and Extrapolation—What procedures should be used to evaluate whether humans are at risk from environmental exposures?

Test-Strategy Uncertainty—How can the overall uncertainty in the testing strategy be best evaluated?

---

be missed if the new assays were used alone and will compel the development of assays to address these gaps. Surveillance and biomonitoring of human populations would also begin during Phase III. Finally, the validated assays would be assembled into panels in Phase IV for use in place of identified traditional toxicity tests.

Validation will be a critical component of the research and development phases. Establishing the validity of any new toxicity assay can be a formidable process—expensive, time-consuming, and logistically and technically demanding. For several reasons, validation will be especially challenging for the mechanistically based tests envisioned by the committee. First, the test results to be generated in the new paradigm depart from the traditional data used by regulatory agencies to set health advisories and guidelines. Second, the many new technologies developed will need to be standardized and refined before specific applications are validated for regulatory purposes. Third, because new technologies are evolving rapidly, the decision to halt optimization of a particular application and begin a formal validation study will be somewhat subjective. Fourth, the committee envisions that a suite of new tests will typically be needed to replace a specific traditional test. Fifth, existing guidelines focus on concordance between the results of new and existing assays; the difficulty will be to find standards for comparison that can assess the relevance and predictivity of the new assays. Sixth, because virtually all environmental agents will perturb signaling pathways to some degree, a key challenge will be to determine when such perturbations are likely to lead to toxic effects and when they are not.

A long-term, large-scale concerted effort is needed to bring the committee's vision for toxicity-testing to fruition. A critical factor for success is the conduct of the transformative research to establish the scientific basis of new toxicity-testing tools and to understand the implications of test results and their application in risk assessments used in decision-making. The committee concludes that an appropriate institutional structure that fosters multidisciplinary intramural and extramural research is needed to achieve the vision. The effort will not succeed merely by creating a virtual institution to link and integrate organizations that perform relevant research and by dispersing funding on relevant research projects. Mission-oriented intramural and extramural programs with core multidisciplinary activities within the institute to answer the critical research questions listed above can foster the kind of interdisciplinary activity essential for the success of the initiative. There would be far less chance of success within a reasonable time if the research were dispersed among different locations and organizations without a core integrating and organizing institute to enable the communication and problem-solving required across disciplines.

Research frequently brings surprises, and today's predictions about the promise of lines of research might prove to be too pessimistic or too optimistic in some details. Therefore, the committee recommends that an independent scientific assessment of the research program supporting implementation of the vision be conducted every 3-5 years to provide advice for midcourse corrections. The interim assessments would weigh progress, evaluate the promise of new methods on the research horizon, and refine the committee's vision in light of the many scientific advances that are expected to occur in the near future.

Regulatory acceptance of the new toxicity-testing strategy will depend on several factors. New testing requirements will be expected to reflect the state of the science and be founded on peer-reviewed research, established test protocols, validated models, and case studies. Other factors affecting regulatory acceptance stem from administrative procedures associated with rule-making, such as documenting scientific sources; providing opportunities for scientific experts, stakeholders, and the interested public to participate; and consulting with sister agencies and international organizations. Implementing the vision will require improvements and focused effort over a period of decades. However, given the political will and the availability of funds to adapt the current regulatory system to take advantage of the best possible scientific approaches to toxicity testing in the future, the committee foresees no insurmountable obstacles to implementing the vision presented here.

Resources are always limited, and current toxicity-testing practices are long established and deeply ingrained in some sectors. Thus, some resistance to the vision proposed by this committee is expected. However, the vision takes full advantage of current and expected scientific advances to enhance our understanding of how environmental agents can affect human health. It has the potential to greatly reduce the cost and time of testing and to lead to much broader coverage of the universe of environmental agents. Moreover, the vision will lead to a marked reduction in animal use and focus on doses that are more relevant to those experienced by human populations. The vision for toxicity testing in the twenty-first century articulated here is a paradigm shift that will not only improve the current system but transform it into one capable of overcoming current limitations and meeting future challenges.

1

Introduction

Toxicity testing is approaching a pivotal point where it is poised to take advantage of the revolution in biology and biotechnology. The current system is the product of an approach that has addressed advances in science by incrementally expanding test protocols or by adding new tests without evaluating the testing system in light of overall risk-assessment and risk-management needs. That approach has led to a system that is somewhat cumbersome with respect to the cost of testing, the use of laboratory animals, and the time needed to generate and review data. In combination with varied statutory requirements for testing, it has also resulted in a system in which there are substantial differences in chemical testing, many chemicals not being tested at all despite potential human exposure to them. Furthermore, the data that are generated might not be ideal for answering questions regarding risk to human health. Accordingly, the U.S. Environmental Protection Agency (EPA) recognized that the time had come for an innovative approach to toxicity testing and asked the National Research Council (NRC) to develop a long-range vision and strategy for toxicity testing. In response to EPA's request, the NRC convened the Committee on Toxicity Testing and Assessment of Environmental Agents, which prepared this report.

HISTORICAL PERSPECTIVE OF
REGULATORY TOXICOLOGY

To gain an appreciation of current toxicity-testing strategies, it is helpful to examine how they evolved, why differences arose among and within federal agencies, and who contributed to the process. The current strategies have their foundation in the response to a tragedy that occurred in 1937 (Gad and Chengelis 2001). At that time, few laws prevented the sale of unsafe food or drugs. A labeling law prohibited the sale of "misbranded" food or drugs, but the law could be enforced only on the basis of criminal charges that arose after sale of a product. During fall 1937, the Massengil Company marketed a drug labeled "Elixir of Sulfanilamide," which was a solution of sulfanilamide in diethylene glycol. From the recognition of the drug's toxicity to its removal from the market by the Food and Drug Administration (FDA), it had caused at least 73 deaths. The tragedy revealed the inadequacy of the existing law. FDA was able to act only because the drug had been mislabeled; at that time, an elixir was defined as a product that contained alcohol. If the company had labeled the drug "Solution of Sulfanilamide," FDA would not have been able to act.

As a result of the sulfanilamide tragedy, Congress passed the Food, Drug, and Cosmetic Act (FDCA) of 1938, which required evidence (that is, from toxicity studies in animals) of drug safety before marketing (Gad and Chengelis 2001). Major amendments to the FDCA in 1962, known as the Kefauver-Harris Amendments, strengthened the original law and required proof not only of drug safety but of drug efficacy. More extensive clinical trials were required, and FDA had to indicate affirmative approval of a drug before it could be marketed. The approval process thus changed from one based on premarket notification to one based on pre-market approval.

The FDCA also dealt with food-safety issues and was amended in 1958 to require manufacturers to demonstrate the safety of food additives (Frankos and Rodricks 2001). FDA was given authority to develop toxicity studies for assessing food additives and to specify criteria to be used in assessing safety. As a result of the need for scientific safety assessments, toxicologists in FDA, academe, and industry developed the first modern protocols in toxicology during the 1950s and 1960s (see, for example, FDA 1959). Those protocols helped to shape the toxicity-testing programs that are in use today.

Differences in testing strategies between drugs and foods arose in FDA because of differences in characteristics and regulatory requirements (Frankos and Rodricks 2001). Drugs are chemicals with intended biologic effects in people, whereas food additives—such as antioxidants, emulsifiers, and stabilizers—have intended physical and chemical effects in food. Thus, a drug manufacturer must demonstrate the desired biologic effect, and a food-additive manufacturer must demonstrate the absence of measurable biologic effect. Regarding regulatory requirements, the FDCA requires clinical trials in humans for drug approval; there is no such requirement for food additives. FDA considers risks and benefits when approving a drug but considers only safety when approving a food additive. Thus, differences in approaches to food and drug testing have evolved.

The public has long been concerned about the safety of intentional food additives and drugs. By the late 1960s, concern about exposure to chemical contaminants in the environment was also growing. In 1970, EPA was established "to protect human health and to safeguard the natural environment—air, water, and land—upon which life depends" (EPA 2005a). Over the years, EPA has developed toxicity-testing strategies to evaluate pesticides and industrial chemicals that may eventually appear as food residues or as environmental contaminants.

The 1947 Federal Insecticide, Fungicide, and Rodenticide Act (FIFRA) required the registration of pesticides before marketing in interstate or foreign commerce (Conner et al. 1987). The statute was first administered by the U.S. Department of Agriculture, but authority was transferred to EPA when it was created. FIFRA has been amended several times, but the 1972 amendments transformed FIFRA and gave EPA new powers, such as classification of pesticides and regulation of pesticide residues on raw agricultural commodities. Although registration remained the centerpiece of the act, one amendment required proof that the pesticide did not cause "unreasonable adverse effects" on humans or the environment (Conner et al. 1987). That amendment was largely responsible for the testing strategy that eventually emerged in EPA.

The other critical pieces of legislation that helped to shape the current toxicity-testing strategy for pesticides were amendments to the FDCA. In 1954, the Miller Amendment "required that a maximum acceptable level (tolerance) be established for pesticide residues in foods and animal feed" (Conner et al. 1987). The Food Quality Protection Act of 1996 amended the FDCA (and FIFRA) and "fundamentally changed the way EPA regulates pesticides" (EPA 2005b). Some of the most important changes were the establishment of a risk-based standard for pesticide residues on all foods, the requirement that EPA "consider all non-occupational sources of exposure...and exposure to other pesticides with a common mechanism of toxicity when setting tolerances," the requirement that EPA set tolerances that would ensure safety for infants and children, and the requirement that EPA develop and implement an endocrine-disruptor screening program (EPA 2006).

FIFRA, the FDCA, and the amendments to them are responsible for the current toxicity-testing strategy for pesticides, which typically requires extensive testing before a pesticide can be marketed. The strategy for evaluating industrial chemicals is different. The Toxic Substances Control Act (TSCA) was passed in 1976 to address control of new and existing industrial chemicals not regulated by other statutes (Kraska 2001). Although manufacturers are required to submit premanufacturing notices—which include such information as chemical identity, intended use, manufacturing process, and expected exposure—no specific toxicity testing is required.[1] Instead, the strategy for evaluating industrial chemicals relies heavily on the use of structure-activity relationships.

FDA's drug and food-additive testing programs and EPA's pesticide testing program represent strategies designed to support safety evaluations of chemicals before specified uses. Other testing can occur in response to regulatory concerns regarding environmental agents. For example, EPA sponsors some toxicity testing, epidemiologic studies, and test development to support its regulatory mandates, such as those under the Safe Drinking Water Act. The Health Effects Institute, a joint EPA- and industry-sponsored organization, funds toxicity studies to inform regulatory decisions on air pollutants. As regulatory concerns arise, industry may initiate testing to evaluate further dose-response relationships of important environmental contaminants. The National Toxicology Program (NTP)—which was created in 1978 to "coordinate toxicology testing programs within the federal government[,]...strengthen the science base in toxicology[,]...develop and validate improved testing methods[,]...[and] provide information about potentially toxic chemicals to health, regulatory, and research agencies, scientific and medical communities, and the public" (NTP 2005)—performs toxicity tests on agents of public-health concern. For example, its chronic bioassay has become the gold standard for carcinogenicity testing. The NTP has been instrumental in the acceptance and integration of new tests or approaches in toxicity-testing strategies. It has initiated development

---

[1]For more information on the extent of chemical testing under TSCA, see the committee's interim report (NRC 2006).

of medium- and high-throughput tests to address the ever-growing number of newly introduced chemicals and the existing chemicals and breakdown products that have not been tested.[2] Tests proposed by NTP and others that are alternatives to standard protocols are formally reviewed by an interagency authority, the Interagency Coordinating Committee on the Validation of Alternative Methods, to ensure that they have value in regulatory decision-making.

Another organization that has influenced toxicity-testing programs in the United States is the Organisation for Economic Co-operation and Development (OECD). OECD is an organization that "provides a setting where governments can compare policy experiences, seek answers to common problems, identify good practice and co-ordinate domestic and international policies" (OECD 2006, p. 7). OECD's broad interests include health and the environment. OECD has been instrumental in developing internationally accepted, or harmonized, toxicity-testing guidelines. The goal of the harmonization program is to reduce the repetition of similar tests conducted by member countries to assess the toxicity of a given chemical. Other OECD programs that have influenced toxicity-testing approaches or strategies include those to define the tests required for a minimal dataset for a chemical and to determine the approach to screening endocrine disruptors.

RISK ASSESSMENT

The toxicity data generated by the strategies and programs described above are most often used in a process called risk assessment to evaluate the risk associated with exposure to an agent. The 1983 NRC report, *Risk Assessment in the Federal Government: Managing the Process,* which presented a systematic and or-

---

[2]The NTP's general approach as described in its *Roadmap for the Future* is reviewed in the committee's first report (NRC 2006).

ganized paradigm, set a standard for risk assessment. The report outlined a three-phase process in which scientific data are moved from the laboratory or the field into the risk-assessment process and then on to decision-makers to determine regulatory options.

The *research phase* is marked by data generation and method development, including basic research and routine testing. For any particular risk assessment, the data used may have many sources, including studies of laboratory animals, clinical tests, epidemiologic studies, and studies of animal and human cells in culture. The data may be reported in peer-reviewed publications, in the general scientific literature and government reports, and in unpublished reports of specific tests undertaken for an assessment.

In the *risk-assessment phase*, selected data are interpreted and used to evaluate a potential risk to human health and the environment. The 1983 NRC report described this phase in terms of four components: hazard identification (analysis of the available data to describe qualitatively the nature of the response to toxic chemicals, such as tumors, birth defects, and neurologic effects); dose-response analysis (quantification of the relationship between exposure and the response observed in studies used to identify hazard); exposure assessment (quantification of expected exposure to the agent among the general population and differently exposed groups); and risk characterization (synthesis and integration of the analyses in the three other components to estimate the likelihood and scope of risk among the general, sensitive, and differently exposed populations). Although risk assessment is based on scientific data, the process is characterized by gaps in data and fundamental scientific knowledge, and it relies on models, extrapolation, and other inference methods. The process turns to science policies—choice of mathematical models, safety factors, and assumptions—to fill in data and knowledge gaps. Science policies used in risk assessment are distinct from the regulatory policies developed for risk-management decisions described below.

Risk management moves the original data—now synthesized and integrated in the form of a risk characterization—to those responsible for making regulatory decisions. The decision-makers consider the products of the risk assessment with data from other fields (for example, economics), societal and political issues, and interagency and international factors to decide whether regulation is needed and, if so, its nature and scope.

The 1983 NRC report and later reports (NRC 1993, 1996; EPA 1998) recognized a *planning and scoping stage* in which a host of scientific and societal issues are considered in advance of research and risk assessment. That activity includes examining the expected scope of the problem, available data and expected data needs, cost and time requirements, legal considerations, and community-related issues. The present report identifies some of those considerations and other, public-health considerations as "risk contexts" and underlines their important role in decisions related to toxicity testing (see discussion under "The Committee's Second Task and Approach" in this chapter).

Reviews and critiques of the 1983 NRC paradigm have for the most part focused on the risk-assessment module and its four components. A review of the literature shows considerably less attention to the research module and the risk-management module. The present report focuses on the research module, in which testing is conducted; however, it ventures into some risk-assessment considerations.

THE COMMITTEE'S FIRST TASK AND KEY POINTS FROM ITS INTERIM REPORT

Anticipating the impact of the many scientific advances and the changing needs of the assessment process, EPA recognized the need to review existing strategies and develop a long-range vision for toxicity testing and assessment. The committee that was formed in response to EPA's request and convened in March 2004 includes experts in developmental toxicology, reproductive toxicology, neurotoxicology, immunology, pediatrics and neonatology, epidemiology, biostatistics, in vitro methods and models, molecular biology, pharmacology, physiologically based pharmacokinetic and pharmacodynamic models, genetics, toxicogenomics, cancer hazard assessment, and risk assessment.

As a first task, the committee was asked to review several relevant reports by EPA and others and to comment on aspects pertaining to new developments in toxicity testing and proposals to modify current approaches. Accordingly, the committee reviewed the 2002 EPA evaluation of its reference-dose and reference-concentration process (EPA 2002), the International Life Sciences Institute Health and Environmental Sciences Institute draft reports on a tiered toxicity-testing approach for agricultural-chemical safety evaluations (ILSI-HESI 2004a,b,c), the 2004 European Union report on the REACH (Registration, Evaluation and Authorisation of Chemicals) program, and the 2004 report on the near-term and long-term goals of NTP (NTP 2004). The committee's interim report, released in December 2005, fulfilled the first part of the study.

As discussed in its interim report (NRC 2006), the committee's review of current toxicity-testing strategies revealed a system that had reached a turning point. Agencies typically have responded to scientific advances and emerging challenges by simply altering individual tests or adding tests to existing regimens. That patchwork approach has not provided a fully satisfactory solution to the fundamental problem—the difficulty in meeting four objectives simultaneously: *depth*, providing the most accurate, relevant information possible for hazard identification and dose-response assessment; *breadth*, providing data on the broadest possible universe of chemicals, end points, and life stages; *animal welfare*, causing the least animal suffering possible and using the fewest animals possible; and *conservation,* minimizing the expenditure of money and time on testing and regulatory review.

The committee identified several recurring themes and questions in the various reports that it was asked to review. The recurring themes included the following:

- The inherent tension between breadth, depth, animal welfare, and conservation and the challenge to address one of these issues without worsening another.
- The importance of distinguishing between testing protocols and testing strategies while considering modifications of current testing practices.
- The possible dangers in making tests so focused that they evaluate only one end point in one species and thus provide no overlap to verify results.
- The need for both chemical-specific tailored testing to enhance understanding of a particular chemical's mode of action *and* uniform testing protocols and strategies to enhance comparability.
- The importance of recognizing that toxicity testing for regulatory purposes should be conducted primarily to serve the needs of risk management.

The recurring questions that arose during the committee's review included the following: Which environmental agents should be tested? How should priorities for testing chemicals be set? What strategies for toxicity testing are the most useful and effective? How can toxicity testing generate data that are more useful for human health risk assessment? How can toxicity testing be applied to a broader universe of chemicals, life stages, and health effects? How can environmental agents be screened with minimal use of animals and efficient expenditure of time and other resources? How should tests and testing strategies be evaluated?

In considering those questions, the committee came to several important conclusions. First, the intensity and depth of testing should be based on practical needs, including the use of the chemical, the likelihood of human exposure, and the scientific questions that testing must answer to support a reasonable science-policy decision. Fundamentally, the design and scope of a toxicity-testing approach need to reflect risk-management needs. Thus, the goal is to focus resources on the evaluation of the more sensitive adverse effects of exposures of greatest concern rather than on full characterization of all adverse effects irrespective of relevance for risk-assessment and risk-management needs. Second, priority-setting should be a component of any testing strategy that is designed to address a large number of chemicals. Chemicals to which people are more likely to be exposed or to which some segment of the population might receive relatively high exposures should undergo more in-depth testing, and this concept is embedded in several existing and proposed strategies. Third, there are major gaps in current toxicity-testing approaches. The importance of the gaps is a matter of debate and depends on whether effects of public-health importance are being missed by current approaches. Testing every chemical for every possible health effect over all life stages is impractical; however, the emerging technologies hold great promise for screening chemicals more rapidly. Fourth, testing strategies will need to be evaluated with respect to the value of information that they provide in light of the four objectives discussed above—depth, breadth, animal welfare, and conservation. In evaluating new tests, there remains the difficult question of what should serve as the gold standard for performance. Simply comparing the outcomes of new tests with the outcomes of currently used tests might not be the best approach; determining whether it is will depend on the reliability and relevance of the current tests.

THE COMMITTEE'S SECOND TASK AND APPROACH

For the second part of the study, the committee's statement of task was to build on the work presented in the first report and develop a long-range vision and strategic plan to advance the practices of toxicity testing and human health assessment of environmental contaminants. The committee was directed to consider the following specific issues:

• Improvements in the assessment of key exposures (for example, potential susceptibility of specific life stages and groups in the general population) and toxicity outcomes (for example, endocrine disruption and developmental neurotoxicity).
• Incorporation of state-of-the-science testing and assessment procedures, methods, and approaches, such as genomics, proteomics, transgenics, bioinformatics, and pharmacokinetics.
• Methods for increasing efficiency in experimental design and reducing the use of laboratory animals.
• Potential uses and limitations of new or alternative testing methods.
• Application of emerging computational and molecular techniques in risk assessment. Issues to be considered included the data necessary to validate the techniques, the limitations of the techniques, the use of such methods to identify plausible mechanisms or pathways of toxicity, and the use of mechanistic insights in risk assessments or testing decisions.

To prepare its final report, the committee held six meetings from April 2005 to June 2006. Three of the meetings included public sessions during which the committee heard presentations by staff of several EPA offices, including the Office of Prevention, Pesticides and Toxic Substances, the Office of Children's Health Protection, the Office of Water, the Office of Solid Waste and Emergency Response, and the Office of Air and Radiation. The

committee also heard presentations by persons in other government agencies, industry, and academe.

To develop its long-range vision, the committee identified a
variety of scenarios for which toxicity-testing information would
be needed to make a decision. Some common scenarios, defined
by the committee as "risk contexts" for which toxicity testing is
used to generate information needed for decision-making, are outlined below.

- *Evaluation of new environmental agents.* This category covers
chemicals that have the potential to appear as environmental contaminants. It includes pesticides; industrial chemicals; chemicals
that are destined for use in, for example, consumer products; and
chemicals that might be emitted by the combustion of new fuels or
new manufacturing processes. It would also include their breakdown products. Because of the large number of new agents that
are introduced each year, a mechanism is needed to test the agents
rapidly for potential toxicity. Questions have been raised about
the safety of and risk posed by new categories of potential environmental agents, such as those introduced through nanotechnology and biotechnology. This category would also include those
substances.
- *Evaluation of existing environmental agents.* Many substances
already in the environment have not been evaluated for toxicity.
In some cases, a need to evaluate specific existing environmental
agents may arise from the discovery of a new source or exposure
pathway or from a better understanding of human exposure on
the basis of, for example, biomonitoring data. In other cases, scru-
tiny may be necessary when toxicity is newly recognized, such as
toxicity in a worker population. In addition, the backlog of untested chemicals in commerce requires assessment to ensure that
the chemicals in use today do not pose unacceptable risks at current exposures. Thus, toxicity testing for existing environmental
agents requires a variety of testing approaches, from basic screen-

ing of a huge set of chemical agents to use of specific data generated by new exposure or health-effects information.

• *Evaluation of a site.* In many areas, soil or water has been contaminated by, for example, former industrial, military, or power-generation activities. If a new use, such as the building of a school or office building, is proposed for such a site, a primary goal would be to protect the health of future users of the site. Other goals could include evaluating the risks to neighbors posed by such a site or determining the degree and type of cleanup needed. Sites that are in use also might need evaluation, such as sites of industrial workplaces, schools, or office buildings. Those evaluations almost always involve concerns about exposures to site-specific chemical mixtures.

• *Evaluation of potential environmental contributors to a specific disease.* Many diseases are suspected of having an etiology that is, at least in part, environmental. A higher prevalence of a disease in one geographic area than in another might require decision-makers to consider the role of environmental agents in the disparity. Understanding the role of environmental agents in a prevalent disease can also help to target actions that need to be taken. For example, asthma, which has seen an increase in prevalence over the last 2 decades in Western societies, is now known to be induced or aggravated by air pollutants. That understanding has allowed decision-makers to take action against some pollutants, but other causes or triggers of asthma could yet be discovered.

• *Evaluation of the relative risks posed by environmental agents.* A risk manager might need to choose between different manufacturing processes or different solvents. Consumers might wish to distinguish between products on the basis of their potential risks to children. A proponent of a new chemical or process might wish to show that it has a lower risk in some ways than the current chemical or process. Such decisions might require less complex risk characterizations if they focus on the possible outcomes or exposures to be compared rather than requiring an in-depth understanding of the risks associated with each possible choice. This scenario emphasizes the need for toxicity-testing information to be directly comparable, standardized, and quantifiable so that such comparisons can be made.

Thus, a primary goal of the committee was to develop a flexible toxicity-testing strategy that would be responsive to the different toxicity-testing needs of the various risk contexts outlined above. Another goal of the committee was to consider the powerful new technologies that have become available and will continue to evolve. For example, bioinformatics, which applies computational approaches to describe and predict biologic function at the molecular level, and systems biology, which is a powerful approach to describing and understanding fundamental mechanisms by which biologic systems operate, have pushed biologic understanding into a new realm. Moreover, genomics, proteomics, and metabolomics offer great potential and are being used to study human disease and to evaluate the safety of pharmaceutical products. Those and other tools are considered to be important in any future toxicity-testing strategy.

ORGANIZATION OF THE REPORT

The committee's report is organized into six chapters. In Chapter 2, the committee discusses the limitations of the current toxicity-testing system, the design goals for a new system, and the options considered by the committee. An overview of the new long-range vision for toxicity testing of environmental agents is also presented. Each component of the new vision is discussed in greater detail in Chapter 3. Tools and technologies that might be used in the future toxicity-testing paradigm are described in Chapter 4. Implementation of the new vision over the course of several decades is considered in Chapter 5. In Chapter 6, the committee considers the implications of the long-range vision given the current regulatory framework.

REFERENCES

Conner, J.D., L.S. Ebner, C.A. O'Connor, C. Volz, and K.W. Weinstein. 1987. Pesticide Regulation Handbook. New York: Executive Enterprises Publication.

EPA (U.S. Environmental Protection Agency). 1998. Guidelines for Ecological Risk Assessment. EPA/630/R-95/002F. Risk Assessment Forum, U.S. Environmental Protection Agency. [online]. Available: oaspub.epa.gov/eims/eimscomm.getfile?p_download_id=36512. [accessed March 29, 2007].

EPA (U.S. Environmental Protection Agency). 2002. A Review of the Reference Dose and Reference Concentration Processes. Final Report. EPA/630/P-02/002F. Risk Assessment Forum, U.S. Environmental Protection Agency, Washington, DC [online]. Available: http://www.epa.gov/iris/RFD_FINAL%5B1%5D.pdf [accessed March 11, 2005].

EPA (U.S. Environmental Protection Agency). 2005a. EPA Commemorates its History and Celebrates its 35th Anniversary. U.S. Environmental Protection Agency [online]. Available: http://www.epa.gov/history/ [accessed February 22, 2006].

EPA (U.S. Environmental Protection Agency). 2005b. Food Quality Protection Act (FQPA) of 1996. Office of Pesticides, U.S. Environmental Protection Agency [online]. Available: http://www.epa.gov/opppsps1/fqpa/ [accessed February 23, 2006].

EPA (U.S. Environmental Protection Agency). 2006. Highlights of the Food Quality Protection Act of 1996. Office of Pesticides, U.S. Environmental Protection Agency [online]. Available: http://www.epa.gov/oppfead1/fqpa/fqpahigh.htm [accessed February 23, 2007].

FDA (Food and Drug Administration). 1959. Appraisal of the Safety of Chemicals in Foods, Drugs and Cosmetics. Staff of the Division of Pharmacology, Food and Drug Administration, Department of Health, Education and Welfare. Austin, TX: The Association of Food and Drug Officials of the United States.

Frankos, V.H., and J.V. Rodricks. 2001. Food additives and nutrition supplements. Pp. 133-166 in Regulatory Toxicology, 2nd Ed., S.C. Gad, ed. London: Taylor and Francis.

Gad, S.C., and C.P. Chengelis. 2001. Human pharmaceutical products. Pp. 9-69 in Regulatory Toxicology, 2nd Ed., S.C. Gad, ed. London: Taylor and Francis.

ILSI HESI (International Life Sciences Institute Health and Environmental Sciences Institute). 2004a. Systemic Toxicity White Paper. Systemic Toxicity

Task Force, Technical Committee on Agricultural Chemical Safety Assessment, ILSI Health Sciences Institute, Washington, DC. November 2, 2004.

ILSI HESI (International Life Sciences Institute Health and Environmental Sciences Institute). 2004b. Life Stages White Paper. Life Stages Task Force, Technical Committee on Agricultural Chemical Safety Assessment, ILSI Health Sciences Institute, Washington, DC. November 2, 2004.

ILSI HESI (International Life Sciences Institute Health and Environmental Sciences Institute). 2004c. The Acquisition and Application of Absorption, Distribution, Metabolism, and Excretion (ADME) Data in Agricultural Chemical Safety Assessments. ADME Task Force, Technical Committee on Agricultural Chemical Safety Assessment, ILSI Health Sciences Institute, Washington, DC. November 2, 2004.

Kraska, R.C. 2001. Industrial chemicals: Regulation of new and existing chemicals (The Toxic Substances Control Act and similar worldwide chemical control laws). Pp. 244-276 in Regulatory Toxicology, 2nd Ed., S.C. Gad, ed. London: Taylor and Francis.

NRC (National Research Council). 1983. Risk Assessment in the Federal Government: Managing the Process. Washington, DC: National Academy Press.

NRC (National Research Council). 1993. Issues in Risk Assessment. Washington, DC: National Academy Press.

NRC (National Research Council). 1996. Understanding Risk: Informing Decisions in a Democratic Society. Washington, DC: National Academy Press.

NRC (National Research Council). 2006. Toxicity Testing for Assessment of Environmental Agents: Interim Report. Washington, DC: The National Academies Press.

NTP (National Toxicology Program). 2004. The NTP Vision for the 21st Century. National Toxicology Program, National Institute for Environmental Health, Research Triangle Park, NC [online]. Available: http://ntpserver.niehs.nih.gov/ntp/main_pages/-NTPVision.pdf [accessed March 11, 2005].

NTP (National Toxicology Program). 2005. History of NTP. National Toxicology Program [online]. Available: http://ntp-server.niehs.nih.gov/ [accessed February 24, 2007].

OECD (Organization of Economic Co-operation and Development). 2006. The OECD: Organization for Economic Co-operation and Development [online]. Available: http://www.oecd.org/dataoecd/15/33/34011915.pdf [accessed March 7, 2007].

2

Vision

Make no little plans. They have no magic to stir men's blood and probably themselves will not be realized. Make big plans; aim high in hope and work, remembering that a noble, logical diagram once recorded will never die, but long after we are gone will be a living thing, asserting itself with ever-growing insistency.

Daniel Hudson Burnham, Architect
Designer of the 1893 Chicago World's Fair

The goal of toxicity testing is to develop data that can ensure appropriate protection of public health from the adverse effects of exposures to environmental agents. Current approaches to toxicity testing rely primarily on observing adverse biologic responses in homogeneous groups of animals exposed to high doses of a test agent. However, the relevance of such animal studies for the assessment of risks to heterogeneous human populations exposed at much lower concentrations has been questioned. Moreover, the studies are expensive and time-consuming and can use large numbers of animals, so only a small proportion of chemicals have been evaluated with these methods. Adequate coverage of different life stages, of end points of public concern, such as developmental neurotoxicity, and of mixtures of environmental agents is a continuing concern. Current tests also provide little information on modes and mechanisms of action, which are critical for understanding interspecies differences in toxicity, and little or no information for assessing variability in human susceptibility. Thus, the committee looked to recent scientific advances to provide a new approach to toxicity testing.

A revolution is taking place in biology. At its center is the progress being made in the elucidation of cellular-response networks. Those networks are interconnected pathways composed of complex biochemical interactions of genes, proteins, and small molecules that maintain normal cellular function, control communication between cells, and allow cells to adapt to changes in their environment. A familiar cellular-response network is signaling by estrogens in which initial exposure results in enhanced cell proliferation and growth of specific tissues or in proliferation of estrogen-sensitive cells in culture (Frasor et al. 2003). In that type of network, initial interactions between a signaling molecule and various cellular receptors result in a cascade of early, midterm, and late responses to achieve a coordinated response that orchestrates normal physiologic functions (Landers and Spelsberg 1992; Thummel 2002; Rochette-Egly 2003).

Bioscience is rapidly enhancing our knowledge of cellular-response networks and allowing scientists to begin to uncover the manner in which environmental agents perturb pathways to cause toxicity. Pathways that can lead to adverse health effects when sufficiently perturbed are termed *toxicity pathways*. Responses of cells to oxidative stress caused by exposure to diesel exhaust particles (DEP) constitute an example of toxicity pathways within a cellular-response network (Xiao et al. 2003). In a dose-related fashion, in vitro exposures to DEP lead to activation of a hierarchic set of pathways. First, cell antioxidant signaling is increased. As the dose increases, inflammatory signaling is enhanced; finally, at higher doses, there is activation of cell-death (apoptosis) pathways (Nel et al. 2006). Thus, in the cellular-response network dealing with oxidative stress, the antioxidant pathways activated by DEPs are normal adaptive signaling pathways that assist in maintaining homeostasis; however, they are also toxicity pathways in that they lead to adverse effects when oxidant exposure is sufficiently high. The committee capitalizes on the recent advances in elucidating and understanding toxicity pathways and proposes a new approach to toxicity testing based on them.

New investigative tools are providing knowledge about biologic processes and functions at an astonishing rate. In vitro tests that evaluate activity in toxicity pathways are elucidating the modes and mechanisms of action of toxic substances. Quantitative high-throughput assays can be used to expand the coverage of the universe of new and existing chemicals that need to be evaluated for human health risk assessment (Roberts 2001; Inglese 2002; Inglese et al. 2006; Haney et al. 2006). The new assays can also generate enhanced information on dose-response relationships over a much wider range of concentrations, including those representative of human exposure. Pharmacokinetic and pharmacodynamic models promise to provide more accurate extrapolation of tissue dosimetry linked to cellular and molecular end points. The application of toxicogenomic technologies and systems-biology evaluation of signaling networks will permit genomewide scans for genetic and epigenetic perturbations of toxicity pathways. Thus, changes in toxicity pathways are envisioned as the basis of a new toxicity-testing paradigm for managing the risks posed by environmental agents instead of apical end points from whole-animal tests.

This chapter provides an overview of the committee's vision but first discusses the limitations of current toxicity-testing strategies, the design goals for a new system, and the options that the committee considered. Key terms used throughout this report are listed and defined in Box 2-1.

BOX 2-1 Key Terms Used in the Report

• *Apical end point*. An observable outcome in a whole organism, such as a clinical sign or pathologic state, that is indicative of a disease state that can result from exposure to a toxicant.

• *Cellular-response network*. Interconnected pathways composed of the complex biochemical interactions of genes, proteins, and small molecules that maintain normal cellular function, control communication between cells, and allow cells to adapt to changes in their environment.

• *High-throughput assays*. Efficiently designed experiments that can be automated and rapidly performed to measure the effect of substances on a biologic process of interest. These assays can evaluate hundreds to many thousands of chemicals over a wide concentration range to identify chemical actions on gene, pathway, and cell function.

• *Mechanism of action*. A detailed description, often at the molecular level, of the means by which an agent causes a disease state or other adverse effect.

• *Medium-throughput assays*. Assays that can be used to test large numbers of chemicals for their ability to perturb more integrated cellular responses, such as cell proliferation, apoptosis, and mutation. Because of assay complexity, fewer agents can be evaluated in the same period than with high-throughput assays.

• *Mode of action*. A description of key events or processes by which an agent causes a disease state or other adverse effect.

• *Systems biology*. The study of all elements in a biologic system and their interrelationships in response to exogenous perturbation (Stephens and Rung 2006).

• *Toxicity pathway*. Cellular response pathways that, when sufficiently perturbed in an intact animal, are expected to result in adverse health effects (see Figure 2-2).

LIMITATIONS OF CURRENT TESTING STRATEGIES

The exposure-response continuum shown in Figure 2-1 effectively represents the current approach to toxicologic risk assessment. It focuses primarily on adverse health outcomes as the end points for assessing the risk posed by environmental agents and establishing human exposure guidelines. Although intermediate biologic changes and mechanisms of action are considered in the paradigm, they are viewed as steps along the pathway to the ultimate induction of an adverse health outcome.

Traditional toxicity-testing strategies undertaken in the context of the above paradigm have evolved and expanded over the last few decades to reflect increasing concern about a wider variety of toxic responses, such as subtle neurotoxic effects and adverse immunologic changes. The current system, which relies primarily on a complex set of whole-animal-based toxicity-testing strategies for hazard identification and dose-response assessment, has difficulty in addressing the wide variety of challenges that toxicity testing must meet today. Toxicity testing is under increasing pressure to meet several competing demands:

• Test large numbers of existing chemicals, many of which lack basic toxicity data.
• Test the large number of new chemicals and novel materials, such as nanomaterials, introduced into commerce each year.
• Evaluate potential adverse effects with respect to all critical end points and life stages.
• Evaluate potential toxicity in the most vulnerable members of the human population.
• Minimize animal use.

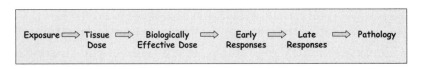

FIGURE 2-1 The exposure-response continuum underlying the current paradigm for toxicity testing.

• Reduce the cost and time required for chemical safety evaluation.

• Acquire detailed mechanistic and tissue-dosimetry data needed to assess human risk quantitatively and to aid in regulatory decision-making.

The current approach relies primarily on in vivo mammalian toxicity testing and is unable to meet those competing demands adequately. In 1979, about 62,000 chemicals were in commerce (GAO 2005). Today, there are 82,000, and about 700 are introduced each year (GAO 2005). The large volume of new and current chemicals in commerce is not being fully assessed (see the committee's interim report, NRC 2006). One reason for the testing gaps is that the current testing is so time-consuming and resource-intensive. Furthermore, only limited mechanistic information is routinely developed to understand how most chemicals are expected to produce adverse health effects in humans. Those deficiencies limit the ability to predict toxicity in human populations that are typically exposed to much lower doses than those used in whole-animal studies. They also limit the ability to develop predictions about similar chemicals that have not been similarly tested. The following sections describe several limitations of the current system and describe how a system based on toxicity pathways would help to address them.

Low-Dose Extrapolation from High-Dose Data

Traditional toxicity testing has relied on administering high doses to animals of nearly identical susceptibility to generate data for identifying critical end points for risk assessment. Historically, exposing animals to high doses was justified by a need for sufficient statistical power to observe high incidences of toxic responses in small test populations with relatively short exposures.

In many cases, daily doses in animal toxicity tests are orders of magnitude greater than those expected in human exposures. Thus, the use of high-dose animal toxicity tests for predicting risks of specific apical human end points has remained challenging and controversial. Inferring effects at lower doses is difficult because of inherent uncertainty in the nature of dose-response relationships. Effects at high doses may result from metabolic processes that contribute negligibly at lower doses or may arise from biologic processes that do not occur with treatment at lower doses. In contrast, high doses may cause overt toxic responses that preclude the detection of biologic interactions between the chemical and various signaling pathways that lead to subtle but important adverse effects. The vision proposed in this report offers the potential to obtain direct information on toxic effects at exposures more relevant to those experienced by human populations.

Animal-to-Human Extrapolation

Other concerns arise about the relationship between the biology of the test species and the heterogeneous human population. Animals have served as models of human response for decades because the biology of the test animals is, in general, similar to that of humans (NRC 1977). However, although the generality holds true, there are several examples of idiosyncratic responses in test animals and humans in which chemicals do not have a specific toxic effect in a test species but do in humans and vice versa. A classic example is thalidomide: rats are resistant, and human fetuses are sensitive. The committee envisions a future in which tests based on human cell systems can serve as better models of human biologic responses than apical studies in different species. The committee therefore believes that, given a sufficient research and development effort, human cell systems have the potential to largely supplant testing in animals.

Mixtures

Current toxicity-testing approaches have been criticized because of their failure to consider co-exposures that commonly occur in human populations. Because animal toxicity tests are time-consuming and resource-intensive and result in the sacrifice of animals, it is difficult to use them for substantial testing of chemical mixtures (NRC 1988; Cassee et al. 1998; Feron et al. 1995; Lydy et al. 2004; Bakand et al. 2005; Pauluhn 2005; Teuschler et al. 2005). Furthermore, without information on how chemicals exert their biologic effects, testing of mixtures is a daunting task. For example, testing of mixtures in animal assays could involve huge numbers of combinations of chemicals and the use of substantial resources in an effort of uncertain value. In contrast, testing based on toxicity pathways could allow grouping of chemicals according to their effects on key biologic pathways. Combinations of chemicals that interact with the same toxicity pathway could be tested over broad dose ranges much more rapidly and inexpensively. The resulting data could allow an intelligent and focused approach to the problem of assessing risk in human populations exposed to mixtures.

DESIGN CRITERIA FOR A NEW TOXICITY-TESTING PARADIGM

The committee discussed the design criteria that should be considered in developing a strategy for toxicity testing in the future. As discussed in the committee's interim report (NRC 2006), which did much to frame those criteria, the goal is to improve toxicity testing by accomplishing the following objectives:

- Provide broader coverage of chemicals and their mixtures, end points, and life-stage vulnerabilities.

• Reduce the cost and time of testing, increase efficiency and flexibility, and make it possible to reach a decision more quickly.

• Use fewer animals and cause minimal suffering to animals that are used.

• Develop a more robust scientific basis of risk assessment by providing detailed mechanistic and dosimetry information and by encouraging the integration of toxicologic and population-based data.

The committee considered those objectives as it weighed various options. The following section discusses some of the options considered by the committee.

OPTIONS FOR A NEW TOXICITY-TESTING PARADIGM

In developing its vision for toxicity testing, the committee explored four options, as presented in Table 2-1. The baseline option (Option I) applies current toxicity-testing principles and practices. Accordingly, it would use primarily in vivo animal toxicity tests to predict human health risks. The difficulties in interpreting animal data obtained at high doses with respect to risks in the heterogeneous human population would not be circumvented. Moreover, because whole-animal testing is expensive and time-consuming, the number of chemicals addressed would continue to be small. The continued use of relatively large numbers of animals for toxicity testing also raises ethical issues and is inconsistent with emphasis on reduction, replacement, and refinement of animal use (Russell and Burch 1959). Overall, the current approach does not provide an adequate balance among the four objectives of toxicity testing identified in the committee's interim report: depth of testing, breadth of testing, animal welfare, and conservation of testing resources.

The committee extensively considered the expanded use of tiered testing (Option II) to alleviate some of the concerns with present practice. The tiered approach to toxicity testing entails a stepwise process for screening and evaluating the toxicity of agents that still relies primarily on test results in whole animals. The goal of tiered testing is to generate pertinent data for more efficient assessment of potential health risks posed by an environmental agent, taking into consideration available knowledge on the chemical and its class, its modes or mechanisms

TABLE 2-1 Options for Future Toxicity-Testing Strategies

Option I In Vivo	Option II Tiered In Vivo	Option III In Vitro and In Vivo	Option IV In Vitro
Animal biology	Animal biology	Primarily human biology	Primarily human biology
High doses	High doses	Broad range of doses	Broad range of doses
Low throughput	Improved throughput	High and medium throughput	High throughput
Expensive	Less expensive	Less expensive	Less expensive
Time-consuming	Less time-consuming	Less time-consuming	Less time-consuming
Use of relatively large numbers of animals	Use of fewer animals	Use of substantially fewer animals	Use of virtually no animals
Based on apical end points	Based on apical end points	Based on perturbations of critical cellular responses	Based on perturbations of critical cellular responses
	Some screening using computational and in vitro approaches; more flexibility than current methods	Screening using computational approaches possible; limited animal studies that focus on mechanism and metabolism	Screening using computational approaches

of action, and its intended use and estimated exposures (Carmichael et al. 2006). Those factors are used to refine testing priorities to focus first on areas of greatest concern in early tiers and then to move judiciously to advanced testing in later tiers as needed. In addition, an emphasis on pharmacokinetic studies in tiered approaches has been considered in recent discussions of improving toxicity testing of pesticides (Carmichael et al. 2006; Doe et al. 2006).

Tiered testing has been recommended in evaluating the toxicity of agricultural products (Doe et al. 2006), in screening for endocrine disruptors (Charles 2004), and in assessing developmental toxicity (Spielman 2005) and carcinogenicity (Stavanja et al. 2006) of chemicals and products. A tiered-testing approach also has the promise to include comparative genomic studies to help to identify genes, transcription-factor motifs, and other putative control regions that are involved in tissue responses (Ptacek and Sell 2005). The increasing complexity of biologic information—including genomic, proteomic, and cell-signaling information—has encouraged the use of a more systematic multilevel approach in toxicity screening (Yokota et al. 2004).

The systematic development of tiered, decision-tree selection of more limited suites of animal tests could conceivably provide toxicity-testing data nearly equivalent to those currently obtained but without the need to conduct tests for as many apical end points. The use of appropriately chosen computational models and in vitro screens might also permit sound risk-management decisions in some cases without the need for in vivo testing. Both types of tiered-testing strategies offer the potential of reducing animal use and toxicity-testing costs and allowing flexibility in testing based on risk-management information needs. Although the committee recognized the potential for incremental improvement in toxicity testing through a tiered approach, Option II still represents only a small step in improving coverage, reducing costs and animal use, and increasing mechanistic information in risk assessment. It still relies on whole-animal testing and is geared mainly toward deciding which animal tests are required in risk assessment for any specific agent. Although tiered testing might be pursued more formally in a transition to a more comprehensive toxicity-testing strategy, it does not meet most of the design criteria discussed earlier.

In the committee's view, a more transformative paradigm shift is needed to achieve the objectives for toxicity testing set out in its interim report, represented by Options III and IV in Table 2-1. The committee's vision is built on the identification of biologic perturbations of toxicity pathways that can lead to adverse health outcomes under conditions of human exposure. The use of a comprehensive array of in vitro tests to identify relevant biologic perturbations with cellular and molecular systems based on human biology could eventually eliminate the need for whole-animal testing and provide a stronger, mechanistically based approach for environmental decision-making. Computational models could also play a role in the early identification of environmental agents potentially harmful to humans, although further testing would probably be needed. This new approach would be less expensive and less time-consuming than the current approach and result in much higher throughput. Although the reliance on in vitro results lacks the whole-organism integration provided by current tests, toxicologic assessments would be based on biologic perturbations of toxicity pathways that can reasonably be expected to lead to adverse health effects. Understanding of the role of such perturbations in the induction of toxic responses would be refined through toxicologic research. With the further development of in vitro test systems of toxicity pathways and the tools for assessing the dose-response characteristics of the perturbations, the committee believes that its vision for toxicity testing will meet the four objectives set out in its interim report.

Full implementation of the high-throughput, fully human-cell-based testing scheme represented by Option IV in Table 2-1 would face a number of scientific challenges. Major concerns are related to ensuring adequate testing of metabolites and the potential difficulties of evaluating novel chemicals, such as nanomaterials and biotechnology products with in vitro tests. Those challenges require maintenance of some whole-animal tests into the foreseeable future, as indicated in Option III, which includes specific in vivo studies to assess formation of metabolites and some mechanistic studies of target-organ responses to environmental agents and leaves open the possibility that more extensive in vivo toxicity evaluations of new classes of agents will be needed. Like Option IV, Option III emphasizes the development and application of new in vitro assays for biologic perturbations of toxicity pathways. Thus, although the committee notes that Option IV embodies the ultimate goal for toxicity testing, the committee's vision for the next 10-20 years is defined by Option III.

The committee is mindful of the methodologic developments that will be required to orchestrate the transition from current practices toward its vision. During the transition period, there will be a need to continue the use of many current test procedures, including whole-animal tests, as the tools needed to implement the committee's vision fully are developed. The steps that need to be taken to achieve the committee's vision are discussed further in Chapter 5.

The committee notes that European approaches to improve toxicity testing emphasize the replacement of animal tests with in vitro methods (Gennari et al. 2004). However, a major goal of the European approaches is to develop in vitro batteries that can predict the outcome of high-dose testing in animals. The committee distinguishes those in vitro tests from the ones noted in Options III and IV. In vitro studies promise to provide more mechanistic information and to allow more extensive and more rapid determinations of biologic perturbations that are directly relevant to human biology and exposures.

OVERVIEW OF COMMITTEE'S LONG-RANGE
VISION FOR TOXICITY TESTING

The framework outlined in Figure 2-2 forms the basis of the committee's vision for toxicity testing in the 21st century. The figure indicates that the initial perturbations of cell-signaling motifs, genetic circuits, and cellular-response networks are obligatory changes related to chemical exposure that might eventually result in disease. The consequences of a biologic perturbation depend on the magnitude of the perturbation, which is related to the dose, the timing and duration of the perturbation, and the susceptibility of the host. Accordingly, at low doses, many biologic systems may function normally within their homeostatic limits. At somewhat higher doses, clear biologic responses occur. They may be successfully handled with adaptation, although some susceptible people may respond. A more intense or persistent perturbation may overwhelm the capacity of the system to adapt and lead to tissue injury and possibly to adverse health effects.

In this framework, the goals of toxicity testing are to identify critical pathways that when perturbed can lead to adverse health outcomes and to evaluate the host susceptibility to understand the effects of perturbations on human populations. To implement the new toxicity-testing approach, toxicologists will need to evolve a comprehensive array of test procedures that will allow the reliable identification of important biologic perturbations in key toxicity pathways. And epidemiologists and toxicologists will need to develop approaches to understand the range of host susceptibility within populations. Viewing toxic responses in that manner shifts the focus away from the apical end points emphasized in the traditional toxicity-testing paradigm, toward biologic perturbations that can be identified more efficiently without the need for whole-animal testing and toward characterizing host vulnerability to provide the context for assessing the implications of test results.

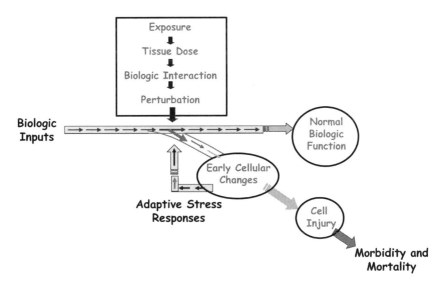

FIGURE 2-2 Biologic responses viewed as results of an intersection of exposure and biologic function. The intersection leads to perturbation of biologic pathways. When perturbations are sufficiently large or when the host is unable to adapt because of underlying nutritional, genetic, disease, or life-stage status, biologic function is compromised, and this leads to toxicity and disease. Source: Adapted from Andersen et al. 2005. Reprinted with permission; copyright 2005, *Trends in Biotechnology*.

Figure 2-3 illustrates the major components of the committee's proposed vision: chemical characterization, toxicity testing, and dose-response and extrapolation modeling. Each component is discussed in further detail in Chapter 3, and the tools and technologies that might play some role in the future paradigm are discussed in Chapter 4.

Chemical characterization involves consideration of physicochemical properties, environmental persistence, bioaccumulation potential, production volumes, concentration in environmental media, and exposure data. Computational tools, such as quantitative structure-activity relationship models and bioinformatics,

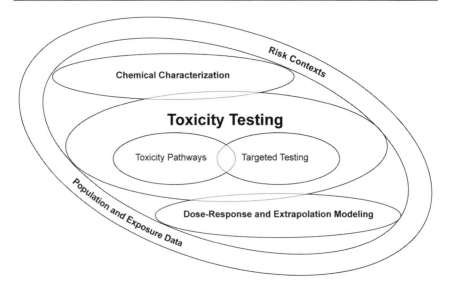

FIGURE 2-3 The committee's vision is a process that includes chemical characterization, toxicity testing, and dose-response and extrapolation modeling. At each step, population-based data and human exposure information are considered, as is the question of what data are needed for decision-making.

may eventually be used to categorize chemicals, predict likely toxicity and metabolic pathways, screen for relative potency with predictive models, and organize large databases for analysis and hypothesis generation.

Toxicity testing in the committee's vision seeks to identify the perturbations in toxicity pathways that are expected to lead to adverse effects. The focus on biologic perturbations rather than apical end points is fundamental to the committee's vision. If adopted, the vision will lead to a major shift in emphasis away from whole-animal testing toward efficient in vitro tests and greater human surveillance. Targeted testing is also used to identify or explore functional end points associated with adverse health outcomes and may include in vivo metabolic or mechanistic studies.

Dose-response modeling is used to describe the relationship between biologic perturbations and dose in quantitative terms and optimally mechanistic terms; extrapolation modeling is used to make predictions of possible effects in human populations at prevailing environmental exposure concentrations. Computational modeling of toxicity pathways evaluated with specific high-throughput tests themselves will be a key tool for establishing dose-response relationships. Pharmacokinetic models, such as physiologically based pharmacokinetic models, will assist in extrapolating from in vitro to in vivo conditions by relating concentrations active in in vitro toxicity-test systems to human blood concentrations.

At each step, population-based data and human-exposure information should be considered. For example, human biomonitoring and surveillance can provide data on exposure to environmental agents, host susceptibility, and biologic change that will be key for dose-response and extrapolation modeling. Throughout, the information needs for risk-management decision-making must be borne in mind because they will to a great extent guide the nature of the testing required. Thus, the population-based data and exposure information and the risk contexts are shown to encircle the core toxicity-testing strategy in Figure 2-3.

The components of the toxicity-testing paradigm are semi-autonomous but interrelated modules, containing specific sets of underlying technologies and capabilities. Some chemical evaluations may proceed stepwise from chemical characterization to toxicity testing to dose-response and extrapolation modeling, but that sequence might not always be followed. A critical feature of the new vision is consideration of risk context at each step and the ability to exit the strategy at any point whenever enough data have been generated to inform the decision that needs to be made. Also, the proposed vision emphasizes the generation and use of population-based data and exposure estimates when possible. The committee notes that the development of surveillance systems for chemicals newly introduced into the market will be important. The new vision encourages the collection of such data on important existing chemicals from biomonitoring, surveillance, and molecular epidemiologic studies. Finally, flexibility is needed in the testing of environmental agents to encourage the development and application of novel tools and approaches. The evolution of the toxicity-testing process, as envisioned here, must retain flexibility to encourage incorporation of new information and new methods as they are developed and found to be useful for evaluating whether a given exposure poses a risk to humans. That will require formal procedures for the phasing in or phasing out of standard testing methods. Indeed, that process is attuned to the need for efficient testing of all chemicals in a timely, cost-effective fashion.

The committee envisions a reconfiguration of toxicity testing through the development of in vitro medium- and high-throughput assays. The in vitro tests would be developed not to predict the results of current apical toxicity tests but rather as cell-based assays that are informative about mechanistic responses of human tissues to toxic chemicals. The committee is aware of the implementation challenges that the new toxicity-testing paradigm would face. For example, toxicity testing must be able to address the potential adverse health effects of chemicals in the environment *and* of the metabolites formed when the chemicals enter the body. Much research will be needed to ensure that the new system evaluates the effects of the chemicals and their metabolites fully. Moreover, as we shift from a focus on apical end points to perturbations in toxicity pathways, there will be a need to develop an appropriate science base to support risk-management actions based on the perturbations. Implementation of the vision and the possible challenges are discussed in Chapter 5.

REFERENCES

Andersen, M.E., J.E. Dennison, R.S. Thomas, and R.B. Conolly. 2005. New directions in incidence-dose modeling. Trends Biotechnol. 23(3):122-127

Bakand, S., C. Winder, C. Khalil, and A. Hayes. 2005. Toxicity assessment of industrial chemicals and airborne contaminants: Transition from in vivo to in vitro test methods: A review. Inhal. Toxicol. 17(13):775-787.

Carmichael, N.G., H.A. Barton, A.R. Boobis, R.L. Cooper, V.L. Dellarco, N.G. Doerrer, P.A. Fenner-Crisp, J.E. Doe, J.C. Lamb IV, and T.P. Pastor. 2006. Agricultural chemical safety assessment: A multisector approach to the modernization of human safety requirements. Crit. Rev. Toxicol. 36(1):1-7.

Cassee, F.R., J.P. Groten, P.J. van Bladeren, and V.J. Feron. 1998. Toxicological evaluation and risk assessment of chemical mixtures. Crit. Rev. Toxicol. 28(1):73-101.

Charles, G.D. 2004. In vitro models in endocrine disruptor screening. ILAR J. 45(4):494-501.

Doe, J.E., A.R. Boobis, A. Blacker, V. Dellarco, N.G. Doerrer, C. Franklin, J.I. Goodman, J.M. Kronenberg, R. Lewis, E.E. Mcconnell, T. Mercier, A. Moretto, C. Nolan, S. Padilla, W. Phang, R. Solecki, L. Tilbury, B. van Ravenzwaay, and D.C. Wolf. 2006. A tiered approach to systemic toxicity testing for agricultural chemical safety assessment. Crit. Rev. Toxicol. 36(1):37-68.

Feron, V.J., J.P. Groten, D. Jonker, F.R. Cassee, and P.J. van Bladeren. 1995. Toxicology of chemical mixtures: Challenges for today and the future. Toxicology 105(2-3):415-427.

Frasor, J., J.M. Danes, B. Komm, K.C.N. Chang, C.R. Lyttle, and B.S. Katzenellenbogen. 2003. Profiling of estrogen up- and down-regulated gene expression in human breast cancer cells: Insights into gene networks and pathways underlying estrogenic control of proliferation and cell phenotype. Endocrinology 144(10):4562-4574.

GAO (U.S. Government Accounting Office). 2005. Chemical Regulation: Options Exist to Improve EPA's Ability to Assess Health Risks and Manage its Chemical Review Program. GAO-05-458. U.S. Government Accounting Office, Washington, DC. June 2005 [online]. Available: http://www.gao.gov/new.items/d05458.pdf [accessed March 8, 2007].

Gennari, A., C. van den Berghe, S. Casati, J. Castell, C. Clemedson, S. Coecke, A. Colombo, R. Curren, G. Dal Negro, A. Goldberg, C. Gosmore, T. Hartung, I. Langezaal, I. Lessigiarska, W. Maas, I. Mangelsdorf, R. Parchment, P. Prieto, J.R. Sintes, M. Ryan, G. Schmuck, K. Stitzel, W. Stokes, J.A. Vericat, L. Gribaldo. 2004. Strategies to replace in vivo acute systemic toxicity testing. The report and recommendations of ECVAM Workshop 50. Altern. Lab. Anim. 32(4):437-459.

Haney, S.A., P. LaPan, J. Pan, and J. Zhang. 2006. High-content screening moves to the front of the line. Drug Discov. Today 11(19-20):889-894.

Inglese, J. 2002. Expanding the HTS paradigm. Drug Discov. Today 7(Suppl. 18):S105-S106.

Inglese, J., D.S. Auld, A. Jadhav, R.L. Johnson, A. Simeonov, A. Yasgar, W. Zheng, and C.P. Austin. 2006. Quantitative high-throughput screening: A titration-based approach that efficiently identifies biological activities in large chemical libraries. Proc. Natl. Acad. Sci. U.S.A. 103(31):11473-11478.

Landers, J.P., and T.C. Spelsberg. 1992. New concepts in steroid hormone action: Transcription factors, proto-oncogenes, and the cascade model for steroid regulation of gene expression. Crit. Rev. Eukaryot. Gene Expr. 2(1):19-63.

Lydy, M., J. Belden, C. Wheelock, B. Hammock, and D. Denton. 2004. Challenges in regulating pesticide mixtures. Ecology and Society 9(6):1-6.

Nel, A., T. Xia, L. Madler, and N. Li. 2006. Toxic potential of materials at the nanolevel. Science 311(5761):622-627.

NRC (National Research Council). 1977. Drinking Water and Health, Vol. 1. Washington, DC: National Academy Press.

NRC (National Research Council). 1988. Complex Mixtures: Methods for In Vivo Toxicity Testing. Washington, DC: National Academy Press.

NRC (National Research Council). 2006. Toxicity Testing for Assessment of Environmental Agents: Interim Report. Washington, DC: The National Academies Press.

Pauluhn, J. 2005. Overview of inhalation exposure techniques: Strengths and weaknesses. Exp. Toxicol. Pathol. 57(Suppl. 1):111-128.

Ptacek, T., and S.M. Sell. 2005. A tiered approach to comparative genomics. Brief Funct. Genomic Proteomic. 4(2):178-185.

Roberts, S.A. 2001. High-throughput screening approaches for investigating drug metabolism and pharmacokinetics. Xenobiotica 31(8-9):557-589.

Rochette-Egly, C. 2003. Nuclear receptors: Integration of multiple signaling pathways through phosphorylation. Cell. Signal. 15(4):355-366.

Russell, W.M.S., and R.L. Burch. 1959. The Principles of Humane Experimental Technique. London: Methuen.

Spielmann, H. 2005. Predicting the risk of developmental toxicity from in vitro assays. Toxicol. Appl. Pharmacol. 207(Suppl. 2):375-380.

Stavanja, M.S., P.H. Ayres, D.R. Meckley, E.R. Bombick, M.F. Borgerding, M.J. Morton, C.D. Garner, D.H. Pence, and J.E. Swauger. 2006. Safety assessment of high fructose corn syrup (HFCS) as an ingredient added to cigarette tobacco. Exp. Toxicol. Pathol. 57(4):267-281.

Stephens, S.M., and J. Rung. 2006. Advances in systems biology: Measurement, modeling and representation. Curr. Opin. Drug Discov. Devel. 9(2):240-250.

Thummel, C.S. 2002. Ecdysone-regulated puff genes 2000. Insect Biochem. Mol. Biol. 32(2):113-120.

Teuschler, L., J. Klaunig, E. Carney, J. Chambers, R. Conolly, C. Gennings, J. Giesy, R. Hertzberg, C. Klaassen, R. Kode, D. Paustenbach, and R. Yang. 2005. Support of Science-Based Decisions Concerning the Evaluation of the Toxicology of Mixtures: A New Beginning. Charting the Future: Building the Scientific Foundation for Mixtures Joint Toxicity and Risk Assessment, February 16–17, 2005, Atlanta, GA, Society in Toxicology Sponsored Meeting: Contemporary Concepts In Toxicology [online]. Available: http://www.toxicology.org/ai/meet/MixturesWhitePapers.doc [accessed Feb. 9, 2007].

Xiao, G.G., M. Wang, N. Li, J.A. Loo, and A.E. Nel. 2003. Use of proteomics to demonstrate a hierarchical oxidative stress response to diesel exhaust particle chemicals in a macrophage cell line. J. Biol. Chem. 278(50):50781-50790.

Yokota, F., G. Gray, J.K. Hammitt, and K.M. Thompson. 2004. Tiered chemical testing: A value of information approach. Risk Anal. 24(6):1625-1639.

3

Components of the Vision

The committee foresees pervasive changes in toxicity testing and in interpretive risk-assessment activities. The current approach to toxicity testing focuses on predicting adverse effects in humans on the basis of studies of apical end points in whole-animal tests. In the committee's vision, in vitro mechanistic tests provide rapid evaluations of large numbers of chemicals, greatly reduced live-animal use, and results potentially more relevant to human biology and human exposures. As discussed in Chapter 2, toxicity testing can be increasingly reconfigured with the accrual of better understanding of biologic pathways perturbed by toxicants and of the signaling networks that control activation of the pathways. The use of systems-biology approaches that integrate responses over multiple levels from molecules to organs will enable a more holistic view of biologic processes, including an understanding of the relationship between perturbations in toxicity pathways and consequences for cell and organism function. The central premise of the committee's vision is that toxicant-induced responses can be quantified with appropriate cellular assays and that empirical or mechanistic models of pathway perturbations can be used as the basis of environmental decision-making. Combining a fundamental understanding of cellular responses to toxicants with knowledge of tissue dosimetry in cell systems and in exposed human populations will provide a suite of tools to permit more accurate predictions of conditions under which humans are expected to show pathway perturbations by toxicant exposure. The institutional and infrastructural changes required to achieve the committee's vision will include changes in the types of tests that support toxicity testing and how toxicity, mechanistic information, and epidemiologic data are used in regulatory decision-making. The regulatory transition from the current emphasis on apical end-point toxicity tests to reliance on perturbations of toxicity pathways will raise many issues. The challenges to implementation and a strategy to implement the vision are discussed in Chapter 5.

This chapter discusses individual components of the vision: chemical characterization (component A), toxicity testing (component B), dose-response and extrapolation modeling (component C), population-based and human exposure data (component D), and risk contexts (component E). Component B is composed of a toxicity-pathway component and a limited targeted-testing component. The toxicity-pathway component will be increasingly dominant as more and more high-throughput toxicity-pathway assays are developed and validated. Surveillance and biomonitoring data will be needed to understand the effects of toxicity-pathway perturbations on humans. Finally, the overall success of the new paradigm will depend on ensuring that toxicity testing meets the information needs of environmental decision-making given the risk contexts.

COMPONENT A: CHEMICAL CHARACTERIZATION

An overview of component A is provided in Figure 3-1. Chemical characterization is meant to address key questions,

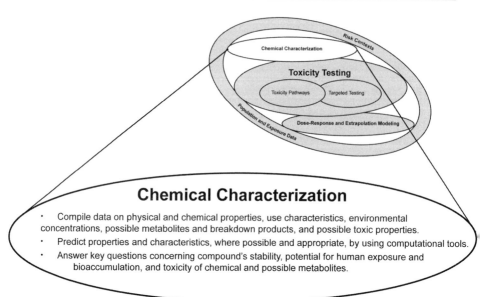

Chemical Characterization

- Compile data on physical and chemical properties, use characteristics, environmental concentrations, possible metabolites and breakdown products, and possible toxic properties.
- Predict properties and characteristics, where possible and appropriate, by using computational tools.
- Answer key questions concerning compound's stability, potential for human exposure and bioaccumulation, and toxicity of chemical and possible metabolites.

FIGURE 3-1 Overview of chemical characterization component.

including the compound's stability in the environment, the potential for human exposure, the likely routes of exposure, the potential for bioaccumulation, the likely routes of metabolism, and the likely toxicity of the compound and possible metabolites based on chemical structure or physical or chemical characteristics. Thus, data would be collected on physical and chemical properties, use characteristics, possible environmental concentrations, possible metabolites and breakdown products, initial molecular interactions of compounds and metabolites with cellular components, and possible toxic properties. A variety of computational methods might be used to predict those properties when data are not available. Decisions could be made after chemical characterization about further testing that might or might not be required. For example, if a chemical were produced in such a manner that it would never reach the environment or were sufficiently persistent and biologically reactive, further toxicity evaluation might not be necessary for regulatory decision-making. Moreover, computational tools for estimating biologic activities and potency could be useful in assessing characteristics of compounds during their development or in a premanufacturing scenario to rule out development or introduction of compounds that are expected to lead to biologically important perturbations in toxicity pathways. In most cases, chemical characterization alone is not expected to be sufficient to reach decisions about the toxicity of an environmental agent.

The tools for chemical characterization will include a variety of empirical and computational methods. As outlined in the committee's first report (NRC 2006a), computational approaches that can and most likely will be used are in the following categories: tools to calculate physical and chemical properties, models that predict metabolism and metabolic products of a chemical, structure-activity relationship (SAR) and quantitative SAR (QSAR) models that predict biologic activity from molecular structure, and models that predict specific molecular interactions, such as protein-ligand binding, tissue binding, and tissue solubility. An array of computational tools is available to calculate physical and chemical properties (Volarath et al. 2004; Olsen et al. 2006; Grimme et al. 2007; Balazs 2007). Tools for assessing metabolic fate and biologic activity are continually evolving, and many of the more accurate and refined examples rely on proprietary technology or proprietary databases. Databases that support the most predictive tools may therefore end up being proprietary and substantially different from those available in the public domain. The committee urges the Environmental Protection Agency (EPA) to consider taking a lead role in ensuring public access to the datasets that are developed for predictive modeling and in providing the resources necessary for the continual evolution of methods to develop SAR, QSAR, and other predictive modeling tools.

Many models used to predict hazard are based only on structure and physical and chemical properties and rely on historical datasets. Their reliability is limited by the relevant datasets, which are continually evolving and increasing in size and accessibility. That is, the predictive value of the structure-activity rules will depend on the chemicals in the dataset from which they are derived—their prevalence, structures, and whether they have the toxic activity of interest (see, for example, Battelle 2002). Computational approaches for predicting toxicity and molecular interactions are available for only a small number of end points, such as estrogen-receptor binding, and their predictive value can be low (Battelle 2002). As approaches improve with time and experience and as the datasets available for model development become larger and more robust, computational tools should become much more useful for chemical characterization, predicting activity in toxicity pathways, and early-stage decision-making.

COMPONENT B: TOXICITY TESTING OF COMPOUNDS AND METABOLITES

The long-term vision makes the development of predictive toxicity-pathway-based assays the central component of a broad toxicity-testing strategy for assessing biologic activity of new or existing compounds. The assays will be conducted primarily with cells or cell lines, optimally with human cells or cell lines, and as time passes, the need for traditional apical animal tests will be greatly reduced and optimally eliminated. The overview of component B provided in Figure 3-2 indicates that toxicity testing will include both pathway testing and targeted testing, which are discussed further below.

A period of transition is inevitable because of the need to develop the full suite of toxicity-pathway tests that will be required for a comprehensive assessment of toxicity. Challenges related to the transition from the current paradigm oriented to apical end points to that outlined here are addressed separately in Chapter 5.

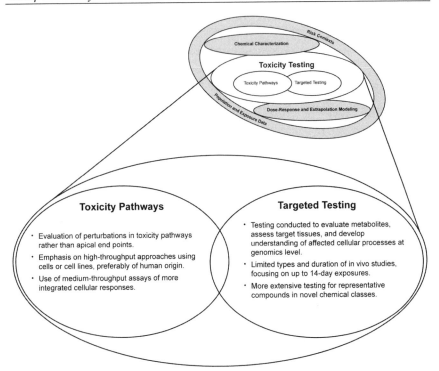

FIGURE 3-2 Toxicity-testing component, which includes toxicity-pathway testing in cells and cell lines and targeted testing in whole animals.

Toxicity Pathways

The committee's vision focuses on toxicity pathways. Toxicity pathways are simply normal cellular response pathways that are expected to result in adverse health effects when sufficiently perturbed. For example, in early studies of cancer biology, specific genes that were associated with malignant growth and transformation were called oncogenes (those promoting unrestrained cell replication) and tumor-suppressor genes (those restricting replication). Both oncogenes and tumor-suppressor genes were later found to code for proteins that played important roles in normal biology. For example, oncogenes were involved in cell replication, and suppressor-gene products normally halted some key part of the replication process. However, mutations (such as those which can be induced by some environmental agents) were found to make oncogenes constitutively active or to cause a great reduction in or loss of activity of suppressor genes.

It is the ability of otherwise normal cellular response pathways to be targets for environmental agents that leads to their definition as *toxicity pathways*. Perturbations of toxicity pathways can be evaluated with a variety of assays, including relatively straightforward biochemical assays, such as receptor-binding or reporter-gene expression, or more integrated cellular response assays, such as assays to evaluate proliferation of an estrogen-responsive cell line after treatment with environmental agents. Cellular responses can be broadly dichotomized as those requiring recognition of the structure of an environmental agent and those occurring because of reactivity of the environmental agent. In the first case, the three-dimensional structure is recognized by macromolecular receptors, as with estrogenic compounds. Accordingly, tests for the structurally mediated responses could be based on binding assays or on integrated cellular-response events, such as proliferation, induction of new proteins, or alteration of phosphorylation status of cells after exposure to environmental agents. In the second case, with reactivity-driven responses, the compound or a metabolite reacts with and damages cellular structures. Reactive compounds have the capacity to be much more promiscuous in their targets in cells, and the initial stress responses to tissue reactivity with these agents may also trigger adaptive changes to maintain homeostasis in the face of increased cellular stress (see Figure 2-2).

Biologic systems from single cells to complex plant and animal organisms have evolved many mechanisms to respond to and counter stressors in their environment. Many responses are mediated through coordinated changes in expression of genes in specific patterns, which result in new operational characteristics of affected cells (Ho et al. 2006; Schilter et al. 2006; Singh and DuMond 2007). Many stress-response pathways—such as those regulated by hsp90-mediated regulation of chaperone proteins, by Nrf2-mediated antioxidant-element control of cellular glutathione, or by steroid-hormone family (for example, PPAR, CAR, and PXR) receptor-mediated induction of xenobiotic metabolizing enzymes—are conserved across many vertebrate species (Aranda and Pascual 2001; Handschin and Meyer 2005; Westerheide and Morimoto 2005; Kobayashi and Yamamoto 2006). Initial responses to stressors represent adaptation to maintain normal function. When stressors are applied at increasingly high concentrations in combination with other stressors, in sensitive hosts, or during sensitive life stages, adaptation fails, and adverse effects occur in the cell and organism (see Figure 2-2).

As stated, the committee's long-range vision capitalizes on the identification and use of toxicity pathways as the basis of a new approach to toxicity testing and dose-response modeling. An important question for toxicity-testing strategies concerns the number of pathways that might need to be examined as primary targets of chemical toxicants. For example, in the case of reproductive and developmental toxicity, the National Research Council Committee on Developmental Toxicology listed 17 primary intracellular and intercellular signaling pathways that were then known to be involved in normal development (NRC 2000). Those pathways and the various points for toxic interaction with them are potential targets of chemicals whose structures mimic or disrupt portions of them. Some of the pathways are also important at other life stages, and biologically significant perturbations of them might result in long-lasting effects or effects that are manifested later in life. As discussed in Chapter 5, considerable effort will be required to determine which pathways ultimately to include in the suite of toxicity pathways for testing and what patterns and magnitudes of perturbations will lead to adverse effects.

Some examples of toxicity pathways that could be evaluated with high-throughput methods are listed below, where the consequences of pathway activation are also noted. Most tests are expected to use high-throughput methods, but others could include medium-throughput assays of more integrated cellular responses, such as cytotoxicity, cell proliferation, and apoptosis. Simpler assays, such as receptor binding or reactivity of compounds with targets (for example, tests of inhibition of cholinesterase activity), also could be used as needed.

• *Nrf2 antioxidant-response pathway* (McMahon et al. 2006; Zhang 2006). The activation of antioxidant-response element signaling occurs through oxidation of sentinel sulfhydryls on the protein Keap1. Some agents, such as chlorine, activate Nrf2 signaling in vitro, and the oxidative stress likely is the cause of irritation and toxicity in the respiratory tract.

• *Heat-shock-response pathway* (Maroni et al. 2003; Westerheide and Morimoto 2005). The activation of protein synthesis by HSP1 transcription factor signaling maintains cellular proteins in an active folded configuration in response to stressors that cause unfolding and denaturation.

• *PXR, CAR, PPAR, and AhR response pathways* (Waxman 1999; Handschin and Meyer 2005; Hillegass et al. 2006; Timsit and Negishi 2006; Li et al. 2006). The activation of xenobiotic metabolizing pathways by transcriptional activation reduces concentrations of some biologically active xenobiotics and enhances elimination from the body as metabolites (Nebert 1994); it can also increase the activation of other xenobiotics to more toxic forms. The toxicity and carcinogenicity of some agents, such as polyaromatic hydrocarbons, occur because of production of mutagenic metabolites by inducible oxidative enzymes.

• *Hypo-osmolarity-response pathway* (Subramanya and Mensa-Wilmot 2006). Cellular stressors damage the integrity of the cellular membranes and activate p38 MAP kinase-mediated pathways to counter them (Van Wuytswinkel et al. 2000). The p38 MAP kinase functionality for the stress responses is conserved across eukaryotes.

• *DNA-response pathways* (Nordstrand et al. 2007). Damage to DNA structures induces repair enzymes that act through

GADD45 (Sheikh et al. 2000) and other proteins. Unrepaired damage increases the risk of mutation during cell division and increases the risk of cancer.

- *Endogenous-hormone-response pathways* (NRC 1999; Harrington et al. 2006). Enhancement or suppression of activity of transcriptionally active hormone receptors—including estrogen, androgen, thyroid, and progesterone receptors (Aranda and Pascual 2001)—leads to altered homeostasis and alteration in biologic functions that are controlled by the receptors.

The biologic revolution now making its way into toxicity testing sets the stage for the design of mechanistic cell-based assays that can be evaluated primarily with high-throughput approaches to testing. The promise of the novel cell-system assays is becoming apparent in advances in several areas: genomic studies of cellular signaling networks affected by chemical exposures, identification of common toxicity pathways that regulate outcomes in diverse tissues, and understanding of networks that control cell responses to external stressors. To ensure the value of results for use in environmental decision-making, the toxicity-pathway assays should be amenable to measurements of dose-response relationships over a broad range of concentrations. Chemical concentrations should be measured directly in the media used in the toxicity-pathway assays when administered concentrations might not represent the concentrations in vitro (for example, in the case of volatile compounds).

Finding new assays for assessing the dose-response characteristics of the toxicity pathways will have high priority for research and standardization. Environmental agents on which animal, human, and cellular evidence consistently demonstrates increased risk of adverse health outcomes could serve as positive controls for evaluation of toxicity-pathway assays. Those controls would serve as standards for the evaluation of the ability of other compounds to perturb the assayed toxicity pathways. Negative controls would also be needed to evaluate the specificity of responses for the key toxicity pathways. For risk implications in specific populations, interpretation of the studies would consider the results of the assays coupled with information on host susceptibility from other human cell or tissue assays and population-based studies. The research needed to implement the toxicity-pathway approach is discussed further in Chapter 5.

Targeted Testing

As discussed in Chapter 2, an integral part of the committee's vision is targeted testing, which would be used to complement toxicity-pathway testing and used in the following circumstances:

- To clarify substantial uncertainties in the interpretation of toxicity-pathway data.
- To understand effects of representative prototype compounds from classes of materials, such as nanoparticles, that may activate toxicity pathways not included in a standard suite of assays.
- To refine a risk estimate when the targeted testing can reduce uncertainty, and a more refined estimate is needed for decision-making.
- To investigate the production of possibly toxic metabolites of new compounds.
- To fill gaps in the toxicity-pathway testing strategy to ensure that critical toxicity pathways and end points are adequately covered.

One of the challenges of developing an in vitro test system to evaluate toxicity is the current inability of cell assays to mirror the metabolism of a whole animal (Coecke et al. 2006). For the foreseeable future, any in vitro strategy will need to include a provision to assess likely metabolites with whole-animal testing. The metabolites would also need to be tested in a suite of in vitro assays. For very reactive metabolites, the suite of assays should include cell models that have biotransformation enzymes required for metabolism. Although it may become possible to make comprehensive predictions of metabolism of environmental agents, any plan to implement the vision here will probably have to rely on some metabolite-identification studies in whole animals. Another challenge is adequate development of in vitro assays to identify reliably toxicity pathways that are causally related to neurodevelopment and other physiologic processes that depend on timing and patterns of exposure and the interactions of multiple pathways. In the near term, targeted in vivo testing will most likely be needed to address those types of toxicities.

Targeted testing might be conducted in vivo or in vitro, depending on the conditions and the toxicity tests available. In the case of metabolite studies, one approach might be to dose small groups of animals with radiolabeled compound, to separate and characterize the excreted radioactivity with modern analytic techniques, and to compare the metabolite structure with known chemistries to determine the need for testing specific metabolites. Similar studies might be conducted in tissue bioreactors, especially a liver bioreactor or cocultures of cells from human liver and other tissues that might make the studies more applicable to human metabolism. Concerns raised in evaluations of metabolism could necessitate synthesis of specific metabolites that would then be tested in the main toxicity-pathway assays. In the development of the European Centre for the Validation of Alternative Methods, there has been extensive discussion of the challenges of capturing the possible toxicity of metabolites so as not to miss ultimate toxicities of substances with in vitro testing (Coecke et al. 2005, 2006).

Although targeted tests could be based on existing toxicity-test systems, they will probably differ from traditional tests in the long term. They could use transgenic species, isogenic strains, new animal models, or other novel test systems (see the committee's interim report [NRC 2006a] for further discussion) and could include a toxicogenomic evaluation of tissue responses over wide dose ranges. Whatever system is used, testing protocols would maximize the amount of information gained from whole-animal toxicity testing. For example, routinely used whole-animal toxicity-testing protocols could provide mode-of-action information on toxicity pathways and target tissues in short-term repeat studies. They could emphasize measurement of metabolite formation and applications of transcriptomics and bioinformatics; future designs might include other -*omic* approaches as the technologies mature and the costs of such studies decrease. Toxicogenomic studies of 14-30 days could provide tissues for microarray analysis and information on pathology. They would harvest a suite of major tissues, mRNA analysis would be performed, and bioinformatics analysis would be conducted to evaluate dose-response relationships in connection with changes in genes and groups of related genes. mRNA from tissues with evidence of pathologic alterations at high doses might also be examined with the major tissues. Thus, the targeted testing in the committee's vision will not necessarily resemble the standard whole-animal assays now conducted either in the protocol used or in the information gained.

COMPONENT C: DOSE-RESPONSE AND EXTRAPOLATION MODELING

The committee's vision includes dose-response and extrapolation modeling modules, which are discussed below; an overview of this component is provided in Figure 3-3.

Empirical Dose-Response Modeling

As they are currently used in toxicity testing with apical end points, empirical dose-response (EDR) models often describe a relationship between the incidence of the end point and either the

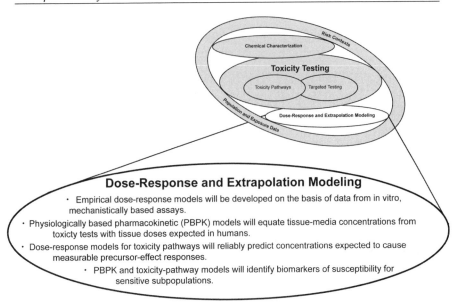

FIGURE 3-3 Overview of dose-response and extrapolation modeling component.

dose given to the animal or the concentration of the environmental agent or its metabolite in the target tissue. In the long-
range vision, the committee believes that EDR models will be developed for environmental agents primarily on the basis of data
from in vitro, mechanistically based assays described in component B. The EDR models would describe the relationship between
the concentration in the test medium and the degree of in vitro
response; in some cases, they would provide an estimate of some
effective concentration at which a specified level of response occurs. The effective concentration could describe, for example, a
percentage of maximal response or a statistical increase above
background for a more integrated assay, such as an enhanced-cell-
proliferation assay. Considerations in the interpretation of in vitro
response metrics would include responses in positive and negative controls, their statistical variability, background historical

data, and the experimental dose-response data on the test substance. In general, the toxicity-pathway evaluations require consideration of increases in continuous rather than dichotomous responses.

Dose measures in targeted-testing studies conducted in whole animals could also be expressed in relation to a measure of tissue or plasma concentrations of the parent compound or a metabolite in the organism, such as blood concentration, area under a concentration-time course curve, and rate of metabolism. Preferably, the concentrations would be based on empirical measurements rather than on predictions from pharmacokinetic models. The main reason for insisting that the in vivo studies have a measure of tissue concentration is to permit comparison with the results from the in vitro assays.

In some risk contexts, an EDR model based on in vitro assay results might provide adequate data for a risk-management decision, for example, if host-susceptibility factors of a compound in humans are well understood and human biomonitoring provides good information about its tissue or blood concentrations and about other exposures that affect the toxicity pathway in a human population. Effective concentrations in the suite of in vitro mechanistic assays could be adjusted for host susceptibility and then compared with the human biomonitoring data. In the absence of detailed biomonitoring data and host-susceptibility information, predictions of human response to a toxicant will require building on the data provided by the in vitro EDR models and using physiologically based pharmacokinetic (PBPK) models and perhaps host-susceptibility information on related compounds.

Extrapolation Modeling

Extrapolation modeling encompasses the analytic tools required to predict exposures that might result in adverse effects in human populations primarily on the basis of results of hazard testing completed in component B. In the committee's vision, extrapolation modeling would most likely include PBPK modeling to equate tissue-media concentrations from toxicity testing with tissue doses expected in humans; toxicity-pathway modeling that provides an understanding of the biologic components that control the toxicity-pathway response in vitro; and consideration of human data on host susceptibility and background exposure that provide the context for interpreting the modeling results. As stated in the committee's interim report (NRC 2006a), the computational approaches must be validated, adequately explained, and made accessible to peer review to be valuable for risk assessment. Models not accessible for review may be useful for many scientific purposes but are not appropriate for regulatory use.

Toxicity-Pathway Dose-Response Models

Models of toxicity-pathway perturbations need to be developed to interpret results from toxicity tests in a mechanistic rather than simply empirical manner; they should be achievable in the near future. Toxicity-pathway models should be more readily configured than models of organism-level toxicity because they describe only the toxicity pathway itself and the initial chemical-related perturbations that are believed to be obligatory but not necessarily sufficient for causing the overt adverse health effect.

Several models of normal signaling pathways have been developed, for example, for heat-shock response (El-Samad et al. 2005; Rieger et al. 2005), platelet-derived growth-factor signaling (Bhalla et al. 2002), and nuclear factor kappa-B-mediated inflammatory signaling in response to cytokines, such as tumor necrosis factor-alpha (Hoffmann et al. 2002; Cho et al. 2003). Also, a screen for anticancer drugs has been developed by using the Nrf2 antioxidant-response pathway (Wang et al. 2006), and a preliminary

Nrf2 oxidative-stress model has been developed (Zhang 2006) to examine chlorine as an oxidative stressor and to evaluate both adaptive and overtly toxic responses of cells in culture. Toxicity-pathway dose-response models optimally would describe the interaction of chemicals with cell constituents that activate or repress the pathway (that is, control it) and describe the cellular consequences of activation (that is, the cellular responses, usually altered gene expression, to changes in normal control). Box 3-1 and Figure 3-4 illustrate these concepts in terms of the activation of the Nrf2 antioxidant stress-response pathway.

Although the toxicity-pathway models are discussed here as part of component C of the vision, creation of the models would occur as a natural extension of developing and validating the in vitro toxicity-pathway tests discussed in component B. In other words, the committee envisions that the models would be developed for many assays in component B. The committee recognizes that in the near term there will be continued reliance on default approaches for low-dose extrapolation, such as the linear dose-response model and application of uncertainty factors to benchmark doses or no-observed-adverse-effect levels. The application of uncertainty and adjustment factors to precursor biologic responses from perturbations will not necessarily involve the same factors as currently used in EPA risk assessments for noncancer end points.

The committee emphasizes the important distinction between models for toxicity-pathway perturbations and biologically based dose-response (BBDR) models for apical responses. Approaches to BBDR modeling for complex apical responses—such as cancer (Moolgavkar and Luebeck 1990; Conolly et al. 2003), developmental toxicity (Leroux et al. 1996), and cytotoxicity (Reitz et al. 1990; el-Masri et al. 1996)—have focused on integrated processes, such as proliferation, apoptosis, necrosis, and mutation. Experimental studies and biologic and toxicologic research are still

---

BOX 3-1 Example of Components of Signaling Pathway
That Could Be Modeled

In nontoxic environments, antioxidant genes are repressed through inactivation of the transcriptional regulator Nrf2. The cytoplasmic protein Keap-1 binds Nrf2 and sequesters Nrf2 in the cytoplasm, where it cannot activate transcription of antioxidant genes (see Figure 3-4). Nrf2 bound to Keap-1 is then quickly degraded through the Cul3-based E3 ligase system (Kobayashi et al. 2004). In toxic environments, some oxidants interact with thiol groups on Keap-1, causing Nrf2 to be released and translocated to the nucleus. Once in the nucleus, Nrf2 heterodimerizes with a small Maf protein and binds to antioxidant response elements; this leads to expression of antioxidant-stress proteins and phase 2-detoxifying enzymes (Motohashi and Yamamoto 2004).

The negative-feedback response loop has two major portions, each of which could be the target of model development. First, the inactivation of Keap-1 by oxidants and the later formation of the Nrf2-Maf heterodimer are response circuits that can be mathematically modeled to predict low-dose toxic responses. Second, the expression of antioxidant-stress proteins and phase 2-detoxifying enzymes can also be modeled to predict low-dose toxic responses.

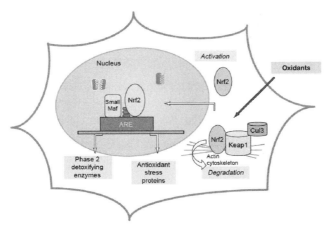

FIGURE 3-4 Nrf2 antioxidant-response pathway schematic. Source: Adapted from Motohashi and Yamamoto 2004. Reprinted with permission; copyright 2004, *Trends in Molecular Medicine*.

required to guide the development and validation of such models. Although toxicity-testing strategies would be enhanced by availability of quantitative BBDR models for apical responses, this type of modeling is still in its infancy and probably will not be available for risk-assessment applications in the near future. Progress in developing the models will rely heavily on biologic studies of disease processes in whole animals and mathematical descriptions of the processes. The committee sees BBDR-model development for apical end points as part of a much longer-range research program and does not see routine development of the models from toxicity-pathway testing data in the foreseeable future.

Physiologically Based Pharmacokinetic Modeling

PBPK models assist in extrapolations of dosimetry among doses, dose routes, animal species, and classes of similar chemicals (Clark et al. 2004). They also support risk assessment, aid in designing and interpreting the results of biomonitoring studies (Clewell et al. 2005), and facilitate predictions of human body burden based on use and exposure patterns in specific populations. The development of PBPK models requires variable investment, depending on the chemical. For well-studied classes of compounds, PBPK-model development might require collection of compound-specific characteristics or statistical analysis to incorporate descriptions of human variability and to describe uncertainty (see, for example, Bois et al. 1996; Fouchecourt et al. 2001; Poulin and Theil 2002; Theil et al. 2003). For less well-studied classes of chemicals, model development might require collection of time-course data on tissue concentrations (see, for example, Sarangapani et al. 2002). Validation of existing models is an important consideration. The possibility of studying the pharmacokinetics of low concentrations in environmentally or occupationally exposed humans provides many opportunities for checking the validity of PBPK models. Advances in analytic chemistry permit kinetic studies at extremely low doses that enable opportunities for such studies.

In the future, QSAR should allow estimation of such parameters as blood-tissue partitioning, metabolic rate constants, and tissue binding and could give rise to predictive PBPK models validated with a minimal research investment in targeted studies in test animals. The goal of developing predictive PBPK models dates back to efforts to develop in vitro tools to measure model parameters or to develop QSAR models to predict model parameters on the basis of physical and chemical characteristics or properties (Gargas et al. 1988, 1989).

COMPONENT D: POPULATION-BASED AND HUMAN EXPOSURE DATA

Population-based and human exposure data will be crucial components of the new toxicity-testing strategy. They will be critical for selecting doses in in vitro and targeted in vivo testing, for interpreting and extrapolating from high-throughput test results, for identifying and understanding toxicity pathways, and for identifying toxic chemical hazards. Figure 3-5 provides an overview of component D, and the following sections discuss how population-based and exposure data can be integrated with toxicity testing.

Population-Based Data and the Toxicity-Testing Strategy

The new toxicity-testing strategy emphasizes the collection of data on the fundamental biologic events involved in the activation of toxicity pathways after exposure to environmental agents. The

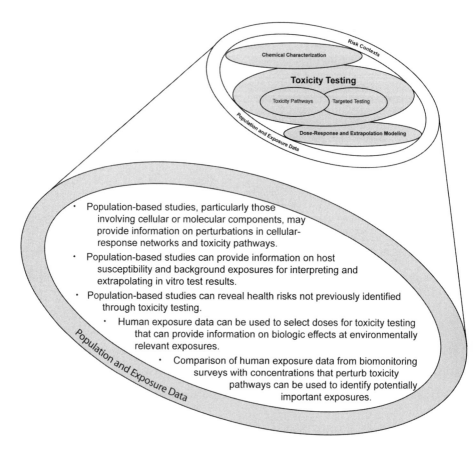

FIGURE 3-5 Overview of population-based and human exposure data component.

collection of mechanistic data on fundamental biologic perturbations will provide new opportunities for greater integration of toxicity testing and population-based studies. In some cases, coordination of the tests will be required; interpretation of toxicity-test results will require an understanding of how human susceptibility factors and background exposures affect the toxicity pathway and how those factors and exposures vary among people.

Genetic epidemiology provides an excellent example of the integration of information from toxicity testing in the long-range vision and population-based studies. It seeks to determine the relationship between specific genes in the population and disease. The finding of genetic loci associated with susceptibility potentially can inform biologists of important cellular proteins that affect disease and can uncover novel disease pathways. Toxicity-testing assays can then be designed to investigate and evaluate the finding and the effects of exogenous chemicals on the disease pathways. For example, human studies have provided information on DNA damage in arsenic-exposed people and motivated laboratory studies on cultured human cells to determine specific DNA-repair pathways affected by arsenic (Andrew et al. 2006).

Conversely, as understanding of toxicity pathways grows, specific genetic polymorphisms that increase or decrease susceptibility to adverse effects of exposure to environmental agents can be more accurately predicted. For example, genetic polymorphisms in some DNA repair and detoxification genes result in higher levels of chromosomal and genomic damage based on the micronuclear centromere content in tissue samples from welders occupationally exposed to welding fumes (Iarmarcovai et al. 2005). Although a substantial amount of normal genetic variation has been identified, only a small fraction of the variation may play a substantive role in influencing differences in human susceptibility. Understanding the biology of the toxicity pathways provides insight into how genetic susceptibility may play an important role. Specifically, a toxicity-testing strategy with a mechanistic focus should define pathways and indicate points that are rate-limiting or are critical signaling nodes in cellular-response systems. Identifying those nodes will allow the potential effects of genotypic variation to be better determined and integrated into chemical-toxicity assessments.

Another example of the interplay between toxicity testing and epidemiology is the generation of potentially important data on biomarkers. The committee's vision emphasizes studies conducted in human cells that indicate how environmental agents can affect human biologic response. The studies will suggest biomarkers of early biologic effects that could be monitored in human populations (NRC 2006b). Studying the markers in a variety of cellular systems will help to determine the biomarkers that are best for systematic testing and for use in population-based studies.

Population-health surveillance may indicate human health risks that were not detected in toxicity tests. For example, although pharmaceutical products are subject to extensive toxicologic and clinical testing before their introduction into the marketplace, pharmacovigilance programs have identified adverse health outcomes that were not detected in preclinical and clinical testing (Lexchin 2005; IOM 2007). Food-flavoring agents provide another illustrative example. In 2000, several cases of bronchiolitis obliterans, a severe and rare pulmonary disorder, were described in former workers at a microwave-popcorn plant (Akpinar-Elci et al. 2002). Exposure to vaporized flavoring agents used in the production process was associated with decreased lung function (Kreiss et al. 2002). Flavoring-associated respiratory disease was also documented among food-product workers and among workers in facilities that manufactured the flavoring agents (Lockey et al. 2002). Although the toxicity of the flavoring agents was confirmed in animal studies (Hubbs et al. 2002), their inhalation hazards during manufacture and food-product production was not recognized at the time of product approval. Situations in which toxicity testing is not adequately conducted or fails to identify an important human health risk emphasize the need to integrate population-based studies into any toxicity-testing paradigm and the need to collect human data in a structured manner so that they can be used effectively by the toxicology community.

Human-Exposure Data and the Toxicity-Testing Strategy

Human-exposure data may prove to be pivotal as toxicity testing shifts from the current apical end-point whole-animal testing to cell-based testing. Several types of information will be useful. The first is information collected by manufacturers, users, agencies, or others on exposures of employees in the workplace or on environmental exposures of the population at large. Such exposure information would be considered in the setting of dose ranges for in vitro toxicity testing and of doses for collecting data in targeted pharmacokinetic studies and in selecting concentrations to use in human PBPK models.

Other valuable information will come from biomonitoring surveys of the population that measure environmental agents or their metabolites in blood, urine, or other tissues. New sensitive analytic tools that allow measurement of low concentrations of chemicals in cells, tissues, and environmental media enable tracking of biomarkers in the human population and the environment (Weis et al. 2005; NRC 2006b). Comparison of concentrations of agents that activate toxicity pathways with concentrations of agents in biologic media in human populations will help to identify populations that may be overexposed, to guide the setting of human exposure guidelines, and to assess the cumulative impact of chemicals that influence the same toxicity pathway. The ability to make such comparisons will be greatly strengthened by a deeper understanding of the pharmacokinetic processes that govern the absorption, distribution, metabolism, and elimination of environmental agents by biologic systems. The enhanced ability to identify media concentrations that can evoke biologic responses will help to reduce the uncertainties associated with a focus on apical effects observed at high doses in animal testing.

The importance of biomonitoring data emphasizes the need to support and expand such programs as the National Biomonitoring Program conducted by the Centers for Disease Control and

Prevention (CDC 2001, 2003, 2005). Those programs have greatly increased the understanding of human population exposure and have provided valuable information to guide toxicity testing. In time, biomonitoring will enable assessment of the status of the toxicity-pathway activation in the population. That information will be critical in understanding the implications of high-throughput results for the population and for identifying susceptible populations.

COMPONENT E: RISK CONTEXTS

Toxicity testing is valuable only if it can be used to make more informed and more efficient responses to public-health concerns faced by regulators, industry, and the public. In Chapter 1, the committee identified five broad risk contexts requiring decisions about environmental agents, which are listed in Figure 3-6. Each decision-making context creates a need for toxicity-testing information that, if fulfilled, can help to identify the most effective ways to reduce or eliminate health risks posed by environmental agents.

Some of the risk contexts require rapid screening of environmental agents numbering in the tens of thousands. Others require highly refined dose-response information on effects at environmental concentrations, the ability to test chemical mixtures, or the use of focused assays targeted to specific toxicity pathways or end points. Some risk contexts may require the use of population-based approaches, including population health surveillance and biomonitoring. The committee believes that its vision for a new toxicity-testing paradigm will help to respond to decision-making needs, whether regulatory or nonregulatory, and will allow evaluation of all substances of concern whatever their origin

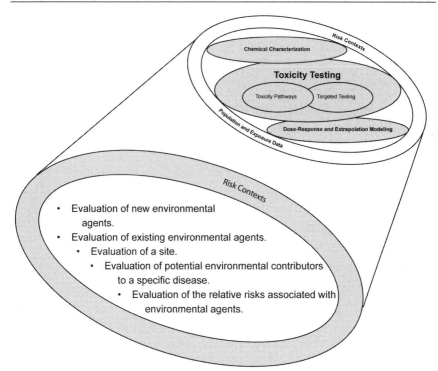

FIGURE 3-6 Overview of risk contexts component.

might be. Specific implications of the vision for risk management can be illustrated by considering the five risk contexts identified in Chapter 1.

- *Evaluation of new environmental agents.* Two issues arise in the testing of new chemicals or products. First, emerging technologies might require novel testing approaches. For example, nanotechnology, which focuses on materials in the nanometer range, will present challenges in toxicity testing that might not be easily addressed with existing approaches (IOM 2005; Borm et al. 2006; Gwinn and Vallyathan 2006; Nel et al. 2006; Powell and Kanarek 2006). Specifically, the toxic properties of a nanoscale material will probably depend on its physical characteristics, not on the toxic properties of the substance or element itself (such as titanium or carbon) that makes up the material. The nanoscale material might be evaluated with new in vitro tests specially designed to identify biologic perturbations that might be expected from exposure to it. As discussed earlier in this chapter, nanoscale materials may require some targeted whole-animal testing to ensure that all biologically significant effects are identified. Second, because many new commercial chemicals are developed each year, there is a need for a mechanism to screen them rapidly for potential toxicity. With an emphasis on high- and medium-throughput screens, the committee's vision for toxicity testing accommodates screening a large number of chemicals.

• *Evaluation of existing environmental agents.* Two issues arise in the testing of existing environmental agents. For widespread and persistent environmental agents that cannot be easily removed from the human environment and can have potentially significant health effects, an in-depth evaluation of toxic properties is important. The committee's vision, with its emphasis on toxicity-pathway analysis, will provide the deep understanding needed for refined evaluation of the potential human health effects and risks. As in the evaluation of new environmental agents, there is a need for effective screening methods so that the potential toxicity of the tens of thousands of agents already in the environment can be evaluated. The committee's toxicity-testing strategy, with high-throughput toxicity-pathway assays, should permit greater coverage of the existing environmental agents that have not been adequately tested for toxicity.

• *Evaluation of a site.* Sites invariably contain a mixture of chemical agents. Evaluation of mixtures has proved to be difficult in the existing toxicity-testing strategy (see Chapter 2). High-throughput assays, as emphasized by the committee, may be the best approach for toxicity assessment of mixtures because they are more easily used to assess combinations of chemicals. Biomonitoring data—whose collection is highlighted in the committee's vision—can be especially useful in site investigations to identify problematic exposures.

• *Evaluation of potential environmental contributors to a specific disease.* Public-health problems, such as clusters of cancer cases or outbreaks of communicable diseases, can have an environmental component. Asthma has distinct geographic, temporal, and demographic patterns that strongly suggest environmental contributions to its incidence and severity (Woodruff et al. 2004) and provides an excellent illustration of how the committee's vision could help to elucidate the environmental components of a disease. First, animal models of asthma have been plagued by important species differences, which limit the utility of standard toxicity-testing approaches (Pabst 2002; Epstein 2004). Second, substantial data are available on toxicity pathways involved in asthma (Maddox and Schwartz 2002; Pandya et al. 2002; Lutz and Sulkowski 2004; Lee et al. 2005; Chan et al. 2006; Nakajima and Takatsu 2006; Abdala-Valencia et al. 2007); the pathways should be testable with high-throughput assays, which could permit the evaluation of many environmental agents for a potential etiologic role in the induction or exacerbation of asthma. Third, environmental agents that raise concern in the high-throughput assays could have high priority in population-based studies for evaluation of their potential link to asthma in human populations, such as workers. The high-throughput assays that are based on evaluation of toxicity pathways can survey large numbers of environmental agents and identify those which operate through a mechanism that may be relevant to a disease of interest, as in the case of asthma, and may help to generate useful hypotheses that can then be examined in population-based studies.

• *Evaluation of the relative risks posed by environmental agents.* It is often useful to assess the relative risks associated with different environmental agents, such as pesticides or pharmaceutical products, that could have been developed for the same purpose. The new toxicity-testing paradigm will provide information on relative potencies established by computational toxicology, toxicity-pathway analysis, dose-response analysis, and targeted testing.

The future toxicity-testing strategy envisioned by the committee will be well suited to providing the relevant data needed to make the critical risk-management decisions required in the long term.

TOXICITY-TESTING STRATEGIES IN PRACTICE

To illustrate how the results of the tests envisioned by the committee may be applied in specific circumstances, two hypothetical examples of environmental agents that may pose risks to human health are considered. The first example is an irritant gas, and the second is an environmental agent that acts by interactions with estrogen receptors. The committee emphasizes that these examples are intended not to recommend definitive procedures for conducting human health risk assessment but simply to show how assessment might be approached. As the research discussed in Chapter 5 is conducted, much will be learned, and new tests and methods to incorporate results into assessments will emerge.

Example 1: Irritant Gas

Toxicity Testing and Empirical Dose-Response Analysis

• Among a larger group of gases tested in multiple high-throughput assays, the agent caused dose-related responses in test assays for glutathione depletion, Nfr2 oxidative-stress pathway activation, inflammatory pathway responses, and general cytotoxicity. Most other human toxicity-pathway tests had negative results, but the test gas was routinely cytotoxic in systems in which gases were easily tested. Nrf2 pathway activation proved to be the most sensitive end point, with an EC_{10}[1] of 10 ppm and a lower bound on the EC_{10} of 6.5 ppm.

- A known hydrolysis product of the test gas—one produced in stoichiometric equivalents on hydrolysis of the gas— produced similar responses in vitro when tested over a thousand-fold concentration range (0.001-1 mM). The test provided a lower bound ED_{10}[1] of 0.12 mM for Nrf2 pathway activation. The hydrolysis product was tested in a broad suite of toxicity pathways and showed little evidence of pathway specific responses, but consistently showed toxic responses at concentrations much above 1.0 mM.

- At nontoxic concentrations, the compound showed no evidence of mutagenicity.

Extrapolation

- *Low dose.* With positive-control oxidants, low-dose behavior of the Nrf2 pathway was shown to be nonlinear because of high gain in the feedback loops that control activation of this adaptive stress-response pathway. A concentration of one-tenth the lower bound on the EC_{10} would not be expected to cause substantial pathway activation. That concentration would serve as a starting point for consideration of susceptibility factors, pre-existing disease in the human population, and possible co-exposures to similarly acting compounds.

- *In vitro to in vivo.* Extrapolation from the in vitro system used a human pharmacokinetic model derived from a computational fluid-dynamics approach. Model inputs derived partially from SAR included reaction rates of the gas in tissues and species-specific breathing rates. The pharmacokinetic dosimetry model

---

[1]EC_{10} or ED_{10} is the concentration or dose that causes a 10% increase in the response or effect over that of the control.

was used to calculate the exposure concentrations that would yield 0.012 mM hydrolysis product (that is, 0.12 mM/10) in the nose and lungs during a continuous human inhalation exposure. The pharmacokinetic model, run in Markov-chain Monte Carlo fashion to account for variability and uncertainty, provided lower-bound estimates of 2.5 ± 0.6 ppm for the lungs and 15 ± 3 ppm for the nose. Sensitivity analysis of the combined toxicity-pathway dosimetry model indicated key biologic and pharmacokinetic factors that had important roles in dose delivery and the circuitry governing Keap1 and Nrf2 signaling.

• *Susceptibility.* Susceptibility would depend heavily on polymorphisms in critical portions of the Nrf2 pathway. People with higher than average Keap1 or lower than average Nrf2 could fail to have an adaptive response to oxidative stressors and could progress to toxicity at lower exposure concentrations. The observed polymorphisms in the human population and sensitivity with pre-existing diseases suggest that estimates arising from the dose-response analysis should be reduced by a factor of 10.

Risk-Assessment Guidance

• The exposure concentration derived from the high-throughput toxicity-pathway screens and the associated interpretive tools could be used in setting reference standards. The assessment would indicate that the concentration should ensure that an exposure would not lead to biologically significant responses to the compound. In addition, the risk narrative would state that this exposure limit should be protective of other downstream responses—such as respiratory tract toxicity—that might be of concern at higher concentrations, because even adaptive, precursor responses are being avoided.

• Estimates of cumulative risk should be considered for situations with simultaneous exposures to the irritant gas and other gases that affect Nrf2 signaling.

Human Surveillance

• Surveillance studies of workers or other human populations potentially exposed to the irritant gas could test for evidence of Nfr2 oxidative-stress pathway activation and inflammatory pathway responses, possibly using induced sputum samples. To evaluate the results, any increases in activation in the exposed population could be compared with pathway activation in control human populations.

Example 2: Estrogenic Agonist

Toxicity Testing and Empirical Dose-Response Analysis

• A large group of commercial chemicals were tested in multiple high-throughput in vitro assays. One of them triggered dose-related activation of estrogenic signaling in receptor-binding assays and increased DNA replication—indicative of cell proliferation—in human breast-cancer cells in vitro. Binding assays for this compound had the lowest ED_{10} values; assay indicators of gene transcription and DNA replication occurred at much higher concentrations. QSAR methods also predicted an estrogenic effect on the basis of a library of tested compounds. All other human toxicity-pathway tests were negative or showed responses at much higher concentrations. The test compound had low cytotoxicity in most screens and produced estrogen-receptor activation at concentrations one-tenth of those which produce signs of cell toxicity.

• A short-term, mechanistic in vivo study with ovariec-
tomized female rats confirmed mild estrogenic action in vivo and
moderate evidence of gene expression for responses in utero or in
breast tissues. Predicted conjugated metabolites of the compound
were without activity in those assays.

Extrapolation

• Experience with estrogen and other estrogenic chemicals
indicates the existence of susceptible populations—such as pubes-
cent girls, fetuses, and infants—that require additional protection
and attention. In addition, chemicals that bind to and activate the
estrogen receptor may act additively with one another. The extrapolation needs to consider the compound uses, subpopulations
that are likely to be exposed to it, other background exposures to
estrogenic agents in these subpopulations, and the estimated tissue dose in pregnant and nonpregnant women, fetuses, and infants.

• Research on estrogen and estrogen agonists reveals that if
receptor occupancy in the most sensitive tissues in susceptible
humans is increased by less than x % by this exposure or any
combined exposure to estrogenic compounds, an appreciable activation of downstream responses or a biologically significant increase in their activation would be unlikely. An alternative assessment would be based on a functional response in a toxicity-
pathway assay, such as transcriptional activation.

• Human PBPK models for the compound would be used to
model absorption, distribution to sensitive tissues, and elimination of active parent compound. The models (for example, Markov
Chain Monte Carlo PBPK model) would be designed to account
for human variability in pharmacokinetics and modeling un-

certainty. The PBPK models could generate a point-of-departure exposure concentration or a daily intake at which there would be less than x % increase in receptor occupancy or less than x % change in transcriptional activation in susceptible populations (for example, fetuses) and in 95% to 99% of the exposed general population. The PBPK models could also provide the blood concentration associated with the change in receptor occupancy or transcriptional activation. That blood concentration could be expressed in units of "estrogen equivalence" to simplify comparisons with estrogen and similarly acting estrogen agonists. Also, on the basis of estrogen equivalence, the models could be used to assess the effects of cumulative exposure to exogenous estrogenic compounds and could be checked against biologic monitoring data in the human population for validity and to ensure that the point of departure is not overestimated.

Risk-Assessment Guidance

• Reference doses and concentrations used in decision-making could be based on a point of departure derived as described above. The reference dose would consider factors, such as susceptibility, that could be altered by polymorphisms in critical portions of downstream estrogen-response pathways or in conjugation with enzymes that clear the compound before it reaches the systemic circulation.

Human Surveillance

• Human surveillance of workers exposed to the compound could detect subtle indications of early effects in humans if they were to occur.

TOXICITY TESTING AND RISK ASSESSMENT

A major application of the results of toxicity testing is in the risk assessment of environmental agents. As illustrated in Figure 3-7, the committee's vision for toxicity testing is consistent with the risk-assessment paradigm originally put forward by the National Research Council in 1983. Chemical characterization and toxicity-pathway evaluation would be involved in hazard identification. Pharmacokinetic models would be used to calibrate in vitro and human dosimetry and thereby facilitate the translation of dose in cellular systems to dose in human organs and tissues. Population-based studies would be used to confirm or explore effects observed in cellular systems to suggest biologic perturbations that require clarification in in vitro tests and to interpret findings in in vitro studies in the context of human populations. All would work together to permit establishment of human exposure guidelines based on risk avoidance, which could be used to enforce scientifically based regulatory standards or support non-regulatory risk-management strategies.

Mode-of-action information is important for informing the dose-response component of the risk-assessment paradigm. A deep understanding of mode of action involves studying the mechanistic pathways by which toxic effects are induced, including the key molecular and other biologic targets in the pathways. Thus, the committee's vision, outlined in Chapters 2 and 3 of this report, is a shift away from traditional toxicity testing that focuses on demonstrating adverse health effects in experimental animals toward a deeper understanding of biologic perturbations in key toxicity pathways that lead to adverse health outcomes. The committee believes that its vision of toxicity testing would better inform the assessment of the potential human health risks posed by exposure to environmental agents and ensure efficient testing methods.

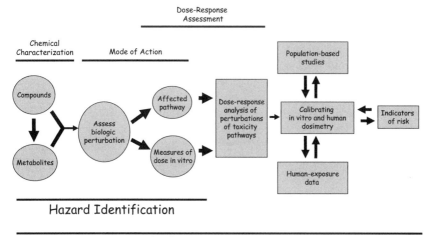

FIGURE 3-7 Risk assessment components. End product is development of one or more indicators of risk, such as a reference dose or concentration.

REFERENCES

Abdala-Valencia, H,, J. Earwood, S. Bansal, M. Jansen, G. Babcock, B. Garvy, M. Wills-Karp, and J.M. Cook-Mills. 2007. Non-hematopoietic NADPH oxidase regulation of lung eosinophilia and airway hyperresponsiveness in experimentally-induced asthma. Am. J. Physiol. Lung Cell Mol. Physiol. 292(5):L1111-L1125.

Akpinar-Elci, M., R. Kanwal, and K. Kreiss. 2002. Bronchiolitis obliterans syndrome in popcorn plant workers. Am. J. Respir. Crit. Care Med. 165:A526.

Andrew, A.S., J.L. Burgess, M.M. Meza, E. Demidenko, M.G. Waugh, J.W. Hamilton, and M.R. Karagas. 2006. Arsenic exposure is associated with decreased DNA repair in vitro and in individuals exposed to drinking water arsenic. Environ. Health Perspect. 114(8):1193-1198.

Aranda, A., and A. Pascual. 2001. Nuclear hormone receptors and gene expression. Physiol. Rev. 81(3):1269-1304.

Balazs, A.C. 2007. Modeling self-assembly and phase behavior in complex mixtures. Annu. Rev. Phys. Chem. 58:211-233

Battelle. 2002. Evaluation of SAR Predictions of Estrogen Receptor Binding Affinity. EPA Contract Number 68-W-01-023, Work Assignment 2-3. Prepared for U.S. Environmental Protection Agency, by Battelle, Columbus, OH. August 1, 2002.

Bhalla, U.S., P.T. Ram, and R. Iyengar. 2002. MAP kinase phosphatase as a locus of flexibility in a mitogen-activated protein kinase signaling network. Science 297(5583):1018-1023.

Bois, F.Y., A. Gelman, J. Jiang, D.R. Maszle, L. Zeise, and G. Alexeef. 1996. Population toxicokinetics of tetrachloroethylene. Arch Toxicol 70(6):347-355.

Borm, P.J., D. Robbins, S. Haubold, T. Kuhlbusch, H. Fissan, K. Donaldson, R. Schins, W. Kreyling, J. Lademann, J. Krutmann, D. Warheit, and E. Oberdorster. 2006. The potential risks of nanomaterials: A review carried out for ECETOC. Part. Fibre Toxicol. 3:11.

CDC (Centers for Disease Control and Prevention). 2001. National Report on Human Exposure to Environmental Chemicals. U.S. Department of Health and Human Services, Centers for Disease Control and Prevention, Atlanta, GA [online]. Available: http://www.noharm.org/details.cfm?ID=745&type=document [accessed July 25, 2006].

CDC (Centers for Disease Control and Prevention). 2003. Second National Report on Human Exposure to Environmental Chemicals. U.S. Department of Health and Human Services, Centers for Disease Control and Prevention, Atlanta, GA [online]. Available: http://www.serafin.ch/toxicreport.pdf [accessed July 25, 2006].

CDC (Centers for Disease Control and Prevention). 2005. Third National Report on Human Exposure to Environmental Chemicals. U.S. Department of Health and Human Services, Centers for Disease Control and Prevention, Atlanta, GA [online]. Available: http://www.cdc.gov/exposurereport/pdf/third_report_chemicals.pdf [accessed July 25, 2006].

Chan, R.C., M. Wang, N. Li, Y. Yanagawa, K. Onoe, J.J. Lee, and A.E. Nel. 2006. Pro-oxidative diesel exhaust particle chemicals inhibit LPS-induced dendritic cell responses involved in T-helper differentiation. J. Allergy Clin. Immunol. 118(2):455-465.

Cho, K.H., S.Y. Shin, H.W. Lee, and O. Wolkenhauer. 2003. Investigations into the analysis and modeling of the TNFα-mediated NF-κB-signaling pathway. Genome Res. 13(11):2413-2422.

Clark, L.H., R.W. Setzer, and H.A. Barton. 2004. Framework for evaluation of physiologically-based pharmacokinetic models for use in safety or risk assessment. Risk Anal. 24(6): 1697-1717.

Clewell, H.J., P.R. Gentry, J.E. Kester, and M.E. Andersen. 2005. Evaluation of physiologically based pharmacokinetic models in risk assessment: An example with perchloroethylene. Crit. Rev. Toxicol. 35(5):413-433.

Coecke, S., B.J. Blaauboer, G. Elaut, S. Freeman, A. Freidig, N. Gensmantel, P. Hoet, V.M. Kapoulas, B. Ladstetter, G. Langley, D. Leahy, G. Mannens, A. Meneguz, M. Monshouwer, B. Nemery, O. Pelkonen, W. Pfaller, P. Prieto, N. Proctor, V. Rogiers, A. Rostami-Hodjegan, E. Sabbioni, W. Steiling, and

J.J. van de Sandt. 2005. Toxicokinetics and metabolism. Altern. Lab. Anim. 33(Suppl. 1):147-175.

Coecke, S., H. Ahr, B.J. Blaauboer, S. Bremer, S. Casati, J. Castell, R. Combes, R. Corvi, C.L. Crespi, M.L. Cunningham, G. Elaut, B. Eletti, A. Freidig, A. Gennari, J.F. Ghersi-Egea, A. Guillouzo, T. Hartung, P. Hoet, M. Ingelman-Sundberg, S. Munn, W. Janssens, B. Ladstetter, D. Leahy, A. Long, A. Meneguz, M. Monshouwer, S. Morath, F. Nagelkerke, O. Pelkonen, J. Ponti, P. Prieto, L. Richert, E. Sabbioni, B. Schaack, W. Steiling, E. Testai, J.A. Vericat, and A. Worth. 2006. Metabolism: A bottleneck in *in vitro* toxicological test development. The report and recommendations of ECVAM workshop 54. Altern. Lab Anim. 34(1):49-84.

Conolly, R.B., J.S. Kimbell, D. Janszen, P.M. Schlosser, D. Kalisak, J. Preston, and F.J. Miller. 2003. Biologically motivated computational modeling of formaldehyde carcinogenicity in the F344 rat. Toxicol. Sci. 75(2):432-447.

el-Masri, H.A., R.S. Thomas, G.R. Sabados, J.K. Phillips, A.A. Constan, S.A. Benjamin, M.E. Andersen, H.M. Mehendale, and R.S. Yang. 1996. Physiologically based pharmacokinetic/pharmacodynamic modeling of the toxicology interaction between carbon tetrachloride and kepone. Arch. Toxicol. 70(11):704-713.

El-Samad, H., H. Kurata, J.C. Doyle, C.A. Gross, and M. Khammash. 2005. Surviving heat shock: Control strategies for robustness and performance. Proc. Natl. Acad. Sci. U.S.A. 102(8):2736-2841.

Epstein, M.M. 2004. Do mouse models of allergic asthma mimic clinical disease? Int. Arch. Allergy Immunol. 133(1):84-100.

Fouchecourt, M.O., M. Beliveau, and K. Krishnan. 2001. Quantitative structure-pharmacokinetic relationship modeling. Sci. Total Environ. 274(1-3):125-135.

Gargas, M.L., P.G. Seybold, and M.E. Andersen. 1988. Modeling the tissue solubilities and metabolic rate constant (Vmax) of halogenated methanes, ethanes, and ethylenes. Toxicol. Lett. 43(1-3):235-256.

Gargas, M.L., R.J. Burgess, D.E.Voisard, G.H. Cason, and M.E. Andersen. 1989. Partition coefficients of low-molecular-weight volatile chemicals in various liquids and tissues. Toxicol. Appl. Pharmacol 98(1):87-99.

Grimme, S., M. Steinmetz, and M. Korth. 2007. How to compute isomerization energies of organic molecules with quantum chemical methods. J. Org. Chem. 72(6):2118-2126.

Gwinn, M.R., and V. Vallyathan. 2006. Nanoparticles: Health effects—pros and cons. Environ. Health Perspect. 114(12):1818-1825.

Handschin, C., and U.A. Meyer. 2005. Regulatory network of lipid-sensing nuclear receptors: Roles for CAR, PXR, LXR, and FXR. Arch. Biochem. Biophys. 433(2):387-396.

Harrington, W.R., S.H. Kim, C.C. Funk, Z. Madak-Erdogan, R. Schiff, J.A. Katzenellenbogen, and B.S. Katzenellenbogen. 2006. Estrogen dendrimer conjugates that preferentially activate extranuclear, nongenomic versus genomic pathways of estrogen action. Mol. Endocrinol. 20(3):491-502.

Hillegass, J.M., K.A. Murphy, C.M. Villano, and L.A. White. 2006. The impact of aryl hydrocarbon receptor signaling on matrix metabolism: Implications for development and disease. Biol Chem. 387(9):1159-1173.

Ho, S.M., W.Y. Tang, J. Belmonte de Frausto, and G.S. Prins. 2006. Developmental exposure to estradiol and bisphenol A increases susceptibility to prostate carcinogenesis and epigenetically regulates phophodiesterase type 4 variant 4. Cancer Res. 66(11):5624-5632.

Hoffmann, A., A. Levchenko, M.L. Scott, and D. Baltimore. 2002. The IκB-NF-κB signaling module: Temporal control and selective gene activation. Science 298(5596):1241-1245.

Hubbs, A.F., L.A. Battelli, W.T. Goldsmith, D.W. Porter, D. Frazer, S. Friend, D. Schwegler-Berry, R.R. Mercer, J.S. Reynolds, A. Grote, V. Castranova, G. Kullman, J.S. Fedan, J. Dowdy, and W.G. Jones. 2002. Necrosis of nasal and airway epithelium in rats inhaling vapors of artificial butter flavoring. Toxicol. Appl. Pharmacol. 185(2):128-135.

Iarmarcovai, G., I. Sari-Minodier, F. Chaspoul, C. Botta, M. De Meo, T. Orsiere, J.L. Berge-Lefranc, P. Gallice, and A. Botta. 2005. Risk assessment of welders using analysis of eight metals by ICP-MS in blood and urine and DNA damage evaluation by the comet and micronucleus assays; influence of XRCC1 and XRCC3 polymorphisms. Mutagenesis 20(6):425-432.

IOM (Institute of Medicine). 2005. Implications of Nanotechnology for Environmental Health Research. Washington, DC: The National Academies Press.

IOM (Institute of Medicine). 2007. The Future of Drug Safety: Promoting and Protecting the Health of the Public. Washington, DC: The National Academies Press.

Kobayashi, A., M.I. Kang, H. Okawa, M. Ohtsuji, Y. Zenke, T. Chiba, K. Igarashi, and M. Yamamoto. 2004. Oxidative stress sensor Keap1 functions as an adaptor for Cul3-based E3 ligase to regulate proteasomal degradation of Nrf2. Mol. Cell. Biol. 24(16):7130-7139.

Kobayashi, M., and M. Yamamoto. 2006. Nrf2-Keap1 regulation of cellular defense mechanisms against electrophiles and reactive oxygen species. Adv. Enzyme Regul. 46:113-140.

Kreiss, K., A. Gomaa, G. Kullman, K. Fedan, E.J. Simoes, and P.L. Enright. 2002. Clinical bronchiolitis obliterans in workers at a microwave-popcorn plant. N. Engl. J. Med. 347(5):330-338.

Lee, C.T., J. Ylostalo, M. Friedman, and G.W. Hoyle. 2005. Gene expression profiling in mouse lung following polymeric hexamethylene diisocyanate exposure. Toxicol. Appl. Pharmacol. 205(1):53-64.

Leroux, B.G., W.M. Leisenring, S.H. Moolgavkar, and E.M. Faustman. 1996. A biologically-based dose-response model for developmental toxicology. Risk Anal. 16(4):449-458.

Lexchin, J. 2005. Drug withdrawals from the Canadian market for safety reasons, 1963-2004. CMAJ 172(6):765-767.

Li, T., W. Chen, and J.Y. Chiang. 2006. PXR induces CYP27A1 and regulates cholesterol metabolism in the intestine. J. Lipid Res. 48(2):373-384.

Lockey, J., R. Mckay, E. Barth, J. Dahlsten, and R. Baughman. 2002. Bronchiolits obliterans in the food flavoring manufacturing industry. Am. J. Respir. Crit. Care Med. 165:A461.

Lutz, W., and W.J. Sulkowski. 2004. Vagus nerve participates in regulation of the airways: Inflammatory response and hyperreactivity induced by occupational asthmogens. Int. J. Occup. Med. Environ. Health 17(4):417-431.

Maddox, L., and D.A. Schwartz. 2002. The pathophysiology of asthma. Annu. Rev. Med. 53:477-498.

Maroni, P., P. Bendinelli, L. Tiberio, F. Rovetta, R. Piccoletti, and L. Schiaffonati. 2003. In vivo heat-shock response in the brain: Signaling pathway and transcription factor activation. Brain Res. Mol. Brain Res. 119(1):90-99.

McMahon, M., N. Thomas, K. Itoh, M. Yamamoto, and J.D. Hayes. 2006. Dimerization of substrate adaptors can facilitate cullin-mediated ubiquitylation of proteins by a "tethering" mechanism: A two-site interaction model for the Nrf2-Keap1 complex. J. Biol. Chem. 281(34):24756-24768.

Moolgavkar, S.H. and G. Luebeck. 1990. Two-event model for carcinogenesis: Biological, mathematical, and statistical considerations. Risk Anal. 10(2):323-341.

Motohashi, H., and M. Yamamoto. 2004. Nrf2-Keap1 defines a physiologically important stress response mechanism. Trends Mol. Med. 10(11):549-557.

Nakajima, H., and K. Takatsu. 2006. Role of cytokines in allergic airway inflammation. Int. Arch. Allergy Immunol. 142(4):265-273.

Nebert, D.W. 1994. Drug-metabolizing enzymes in ligand-modulated transcription. Biochem. Pharmacol. 47(1):25-37.

Nel, A., T. Xia, L. Madler, and N. Li. 2006. Toxic potential of materials at the nanolevel. Science 311(5761):622-627.

Nordstrand L.M., J. Ringvoll, E. Larsen, and A. Klungland. 2007. Genome instability and DNA damage accumulation in gene-targeted mice. Neuroscience 145(4):1309-1317.

NRC (National Research Council). 1999. Hormonally Active Agents in the Environment. Washington, DC: National Academy Press.

NRC (National Research Council). 2000. Scientific Frontiers in Developmental Toxicology and Risk Assessment. Washington, DC: National Academy Press.

NRC (National Research Council). 2006a. Toxicity Testing for Assessment of Environmental Agents: Interim Report. Washington, DC: The National Academies Press.

NRC (National Research Council). 2006b. Human Biomonitoring for Environmental Chemicals. Washington, DC: The National Academies Press.

Olsen, L., P. Rydberg, T.H. Rod, and U. Ryde. 2006. Prediction of activation energies for hydrogen abstraction by cytochrome p450. J. Med. Chem. 49(22):6489-6499.

Pabst, R. 2002. Animal models for asthma: Controversial aspects and unsolved problems. Pathobiology 70(5):252-254.

Pandya, R.J., G. Solomon, A. Kinner, and J.R. Balmes. 2002. Diesel exhaust and asthma: Hypotheses and molecular mechanisms of action. Environ. Health Perspect. 110(Suppl. 1):103-112.

Poulin, P., and F.P. Theil. 2002. Prediction of pharmacokinetics prior to in vivo studies. II. Generic physiologically based pharmacokinetic models of drug disposition. J. Pharm. Sci. 91(5):1358-1370.

Powell, M.C., and M.S. Kanarek. 2006. Nanomaterial health effects-Part 1: Background and current knowledge. WMJ 105(2):16-20.

Reitz, R.H., A.L. Mendrala, R.A. Corley, J.F. Quast, M.L. Gargas, M.E. Andersen, D.A. Staats, and R.B. Conolly. 1990. Estimating the risk of liver cancer associated with human exposures to chloroform using physiologically based pharmacokinetic modeling. Toxicol. Appl. Pharmacol. 105(3):443-459.

Rieger, T.R., R.I. Morimoto, and V. Hatzimanikatis. 2005. Mathematical modeling of the eukaryotic heat-shock response: Dynamics of the hsp70 promoter. Biophys. J. 88(3):1646-1658.

Sarangapani, R., J. Teeguarden, K.P. Plotzke, J.M. McKim, Jr., and M.E. Andersen. 2002. Dose-response modeling of cytochrome p450 induction by rats by octamethylcyclotetrasiloxane. Toxicol. Sci. 67(2):159-172.

Schilter, B., M. Marin-Kuan, T. Delatour, S. Nestler, P. Mantle, and C. Cavin. 2006. Ochratoxin A: Potential epigenetic mechanisms of toxicity and carcinogenicity. Food Addit. Contam. 22(Suppl. 1):88-93.

Sheikh, M.S., M.C. Hollander, and A.J. Fornance, Jr. 2000. Role of Gadd45 in apoptosis. Biochem. Pharmacol. 59(1):43-45.

Singh, K.P., and J.W. DuMond, Jr. 2007. Genetic and epigenetic changes induced by chronic low dose exposure to arsenic of mouse testicular Leydig cells. Int. J. Oncol. 30(1):253-260.

Subramanya, S., and K. Mensa-Wilmot. 2006. Regulated cleavage of intracellular glycosylphosphatidylinositol in a trypanosome. Peroxisome-to-endoplasmic reticulum translocation of a phospholipase C. FEBS J. 273(10):2110-2126.

Theil, F.P., T.W. Guentert, S. Haddad, and P. Poulin. 2003. Utility of physiologically based pharmacokinetic models to drug development and rational drug discovery candidate selection. Toxicol. Lett. 138(1-2):29-49.

Timsit, Y.E. and M. Negishi. 2006. CAR and PXR: The xenobiotic-sensing receptors. Steroids 72(3):231-246.

Van Wuytswinkel, O., V. Reiser, M. Siderius, M.C. Kelders, G. Ammerer, H. Ruis, and W.H. Mager. 2000. Response of *Saccharomyces cerevisiae* to sever osmotic stress: Evidence for a novel activation mechanism of the HOG MAP kinase pathway. Mol. Microbiol. 37(2):382-397.

Volarath, P., H. Wang, H. Fu, and R. Harrison. 2004. Knowledge-based algorithms for chemical structure and property analysis. Conf. Proc. IEEE Eng. Med. Biol. Soc. 4:3011-3014.

Wang, X.J., J.D. Hayes, and C.R. Wolf. 2006. Generation of a stable antioxidant response element-driven reporter gene cell line and its use to show redox-dependent activation of nrf2 by cancer chemotherapeutic agents. Cancer Res. 66(22):10983-10994.

Waxman, D.J. 1999. P450 gene induction by structurally diverse xenochemicals: Central role of nuclear receptors CAR, PXR, and PPAR. Arch. Biochem. Biophys. 369(1):11-23.

Weis, B.K., D. Balshaw, J.R. Barr, D. Brown, M. Ellisman, P. Lioy, G. Omenn, J.D. Potter, M.T. Smith, L. Sohn, W.A. Suk, S. Sumner, J. Swenberg, D.R. Walt, S. Watkins, C. Thompson, and S.H. Wilson. 2005. Personalized exposure assessment: Promising approaches for human environmental health research. Environ. Health Perspect. 113(7):840-848.

Westerheide, S.D., and R.I. Morimoto. 2005. Heat shock response modulators as therapeutic tools for diseases of protein conformation. J. Biol. Chem. 280(39):33097-33100.

Woodruff, T.J., D.A. Axelrad, A.D. Kyle, O. Nweke, G.G. Miller, and B.J. Hurley. 2004. Trends in environmentally related childhood illnesses. Pediatrics 113(Suppl. 4):1133-1140.

Zhang, D.D. 2006. Mechanistic studies of the Nrf2-Keap1 signaling pathway. Drug Metab Rev. 38(4):769-789.

4

Tools and Technologies

In Chapter 2, the committee provided an overview of its vision for toxicity testing, and Chapter 3 described the main components of the vision. Here, tools and technologies that might be used to apply the committee's vision are briefly discussed. The tools and technologies will evolve and mature over time, but many are already available. The committee emphasizes that technologies are evolving rapidly, and new molecular technologies will surely be available in the near future for mapping toxicity pathways, assessing their functions, and measuring dose-response relationships.

TOOLS AND TECHNOLOGIES FOR CHEMICAL CHARACTERIZATION

A variety of computational methods are available for chemical characterization. The discussion here focuses on structure-activity relationship (SAR) analyses, which use physical and chemical properties to predict the biologic activity, potential toxicity, and metabolism of an agent of concern. All are conceptually based on the similar-property principle, that is, that chemicals with similar structure are likely to exhibit similar activity (Tong et al. 2003). Accordingly, biologic properties of new chemicals are often inferred from properties of similar existing chemicals whose hazards are already known. Specifically, SAR analysis involves building mathematical models and databases that use physical properties (such as solubility, molecular weight, dissociation constant, ionization potential energies, and melting point) and chemical properties (such as steric properties, presence or absence of chemical moieties or functional groups, and electrophilicity) to predict biologic or toxicologic activity of chemicals. SAR analyses can be qualitative (for example, recognition of structural alerts, that is chemical functional groups and substructures) or quantitative (for example, use of mathematical modeling to link physical, chemical, and structural properties with biologic or toxic end points) (Benigni 2004). Key factors in the successful application of SAR methods include proper representation and selection of structural, physical, and chemical molecular features; appropriate selection of the initial set of compounds (that is, the "training set") and methods of analysis; the quality of the biologic data; and knowledge of the mode or mechanism of toxic action (McKinney et al. 2000).

Current applications of SAR analyses include soft drug design, which involves improving the therapeutic index of a drug by manipulating its steric and structural properties (Bodor 1999); design and testing of chemotherapeutic agents (van den Broek et al. 1989); nonviral gene and targeted-gene delivery (Congiu et al. 2004); creating predictive models of carcinogenicity to replace animal models (Benigni 2004); predicting the toxicity of chemicals, particularly pesticides and metals (Walker et al. 2003a); and predicting the environmental fate and ecologic effects of industrial chemicals (Walker et al. 2003b). Among the available predictive-toxicity systems, the most widely used are statistically based correlative programs (such as CASE/MultiCASE and TOPKAT) and rule-based expert systems (such as DEREK and ONCOLOGIC) (McKinney et al. 2000).

There are many examples of successful applications of SAR and quantitative SAR (QSAR) analysis. One successful application of SAR analysis in risk assessment is the modeling of Ah-receptor-binding affinities of dioxin-like compounds, including the structurally related polychlorinated dioxins, dibenzofurans, and biphenyls. Specifically, SAR methods were used to establish a common mechanism of action for toxic effects and in the further development of toxic equivalency factors in risk assessments involving exposure to complex mixtures of those compounds (van der Berg et al. 1998). Other successful applications have examined how structural alterations influence toxicity. For example, toxic effects of nonpolar anesthetics are mediated by a nonspecific action on cell membranes and have been shown to be directly correlated to their log octanol-water partition coefficient (log Kow). However, the polar anesthetics—which include such chemicals as phenols, anilines, pyridines, nitrobenzenes, and aliphatic amines—generally show an anesthetic potency 5-10 times higher than expected on the basis of their log Kow alone (Soffers et al. 2001).

Much effort has been directed toward the modeling and prediction of specific toxicities, particularly mutagenicity and carcinogenicity because of the importance of these end points, the cost and length of full rodent assays for carcinogenesis, and the availability of high-quality data for modeling purposes. Experimental observation has led to the identification of several structural alerts that can cause both mutation and cancer, including carbonium ions (alkyl-, aryl-, and benzylic-), nitrenium ions, epoxides and oxonium ions, aldehydes, polarized double bonds (alpha and beta unsaturated carbonyls or carboxylates), peroxides, free radicals, and acylating intermediates (Benigni and Bossa 2006). The structural alerts for mutagenicity and carcinogenicity have been incorporated into expert systems for predicting toxic effects of chemicals (Simon-Hettich et al. 2006).

A number of structural alerts also have been associated with developmental toxicity. They were identified on the basis of known developmental responses to environmental agents, such as valproic acids, hydrazides, and carbamates (Schultz and Seward 2000; Cronin 2002; Walker et al. 2004). Studies have demonstrated that the presence of a hydroxyl group is required for estrogenic activity of biphenyls; symmetric derivatives are 10 times more active than nonsymmetric ones (Schultz et al. 1998). The relationship between the size and shape of the nonphenolic moiety and estrogenic potency among para-substituted phenols demonstrated the trend of increasing estrogenicity with increased molecular size (Schultz and Seward 2000). Thus, although predictive models for some toxic end points, such as mutagenicity, already exist, more mechanistically complex end points—such as acute, chronic, or organ toxicity—are more difficult to predict (Schultz and Seward 2000; Simon-Hettich et al. 2006).

One final application of SAR analysis is in predicting absorption, distribution, metabolism, and excretion. Qualitative SARs, QSARs, and the related quantitative structure-property relationships have been successfully used to estimate such key properties as permeability, solubility, biodegradability, and cytochrome P-450 metabolism (Feher et al. 2000; Bugrim et al. 2004); to predict drug half-life values (Anderson 2002); and to describe penetration of the blood-brain barrier (Bugrim et al. 2004).

As indicated above, the predictive ability of different models depends on selecting the correct molecular descriptors for the particular toxic end points, the appropriate mathematical approach and analysis, and a sufficiently rich set of experimental data. The ability to adapt existing models continuously by building on larger and higher-quality datasets is crucial for the improvement and ultimate success of these approaches.

MAPPING TOXICITY PATHWAYS

As discussed in Chapters 2 and 3, the key component of the committee's vision is the evaluation of perturbations in toxicity pathways. Many tools and technologies are available that can aid in the identification of biologic signaling pathways and the development of assays to evaluate their function. Recent advances in cellular and molecular biology, -omics technologies, and computational analysis have contributed considerably to the understanding of biologic signaling processes (Daston 1997; Ekins et al. 2005). Within the last 15 years, multiple cellular response pathways have been evaluated in increasing depth as is evidenced by the progress in the basic knowledge of cellular and molecular biology (Fernandis and Wenk 2007; Lewin et al. 2007). Moreover, systems biology constitutes a powerful approach to describing and understanding the fundamental mechanisms by which biologic systems operate. Specifically, systems biology focuses on the elucidation of biologic components and how they work together to give rise to biologic function. A systems approach can be used to describe the fundamental biologic events involved in toxicity pathways and to provide evolving biologic modeling tools that describe cellular circuits and their perturbations by environmental agents (Andersen et al. 2005a). A longer-term goal of systems biology is to create mathematical models of biologic circuits that predict the behavior of cells in response to environmental agents qualitatively and quantitatively (Lander and Weinberg 2000). Progress in that regard is being made in developmental biology (Cummings and Kavlock 2005; Slikker et al. 2005). The sections that follow outline tools and technologies that will most likely be used to elucidate the critical toxicity pathways and to develop assays to evaluate them.

In Vitro Tests

The committee foresees that in vitro assays will make up the bulk of the toxicity tests in its vision. In vitro tests are currently used in traditional toxicity testing and indicate the success of developing and using in vitro assays (Goldberg and Hartung 2006). In vitro tests include the 3T3 neural red uptake phototoxicity assay (Spielman and Liebsch 2001), cytotoxicity assays (O'Brien and Haskins 2007), skin-corrosivity tests, and assays measuring vascular injury using human endothelial cells (Schleger et al. 2004). Many tests have been validated by the European Centre for the Validation of Alternative Methods. The committee notes that the current in vitro tests originated as alternatives to or replacements of other toxicity tests. In the committee's vision, in vitro assays will evaluate biologically significant perturbations in toxicity pathways and thus are *not* intended to serve as direct replacements of existing toxicity tests.

The committee envisions the use of human cell lines for the in vitro assays. Cell lines have been used for a long time in experimental toxicology and pharmacology. Human cell lines are readily available from tissue-culture banks and laboratories and are particularly attractive because they offer the possibility of working with a system that maintains several phenotypic and genotypic characteristics of the human cells in vivo (Suemori 2006). Differentiated functions, functional markers, and metabolic capacities may be altered or preserved in cell lines, depending on culture conditions, thereby allowing testing of a wide array of agents in different experimental settings. Other possibilities include using animal cells that are transfected to express human genes and proteins. For example, various cell lines—such as V79, CHO, COS-7, NIH3T3, and HEPG2—have been transfected with complementary DNA (cDNA, DNA synthesized from mature mRNA) coding for human enzymes and used in mutagenesis and drug-metabolism studies (Potier et al. 1995). Individual enzymes have also been stably expressed to identify the major human isoenzymes, such as cytochromes P-450 and UDP-glucuronosyltransferases, responsible for the metabolism of potential therapeutic and environmental agents. The metabolic in vitro screens with human enzymes are usually conducted as a prelude to clinical studies.

A major limitation of using human cell lines is the difficulty of extrapolating data from the simple biologic system of single cells to the complex interactions in whole animals. Questions have also been raised concerning the stability of cell lines over time, the reproducibility of responses over time, and the ability of cell lines to account for genetic diversity of the human population. Nonetheless, cell lines have been used as key tools in the initial screening and evaluation of toxic agents and the characterization of properties of cancer cells (Suzuki et al. 2005) and in gene profiling with microarrays (Wang et al. 2006). The high-throughput methods now becoming more common will allow the expansion of the methods to larger numbers of end points, wider dose ranges, and mixtures of agents (Inglese 2002; Inglese et al. 2006).

High-Throughput Methods

A critical feature of the committee's vision is the use of high-throughput methods that will allow economical screening of large numbers of chemicals in a short period. The pharmaceutical industry provides an example of the successful use of high-throughput methods. Optimizing drug-candidate screening is essential for timely and cost-effective development of new pharmaceuticals. Without effective screening methods, poor drug candidates might not be identified until the preclinical or clinical phase of the drug-development process, and this could lead to high costs and low productivity for the pharmaceutical industry

(Lee and Dordick 2006). Pharmaceutical companies have turned to high-throughput screening, which allows automated simultaneous testing of thousands of chemical compounds under conditions that model key biologic mechanisms (Fischer 2005). Such technologies as hybridization, microarrays, real-time polymerase chain reaction, and large-scale sequencing are some of the high-throughput methods that have been developed (Waring and Ulrich 2000). High-throughput assays are useful for predicting several important characteristics related to the absorption, distribution, metabolism, excretion, and toxicity of a compound (Gombar et al. 2003). They can predict the interaction of a compound with enzymes, the metabolic degradation of the compound, the enzymes involved in its biotransformation, and the metabolites formed (Masimirembwa et al. 2001). That information is integral for selecting compounds to advance to the next phase of drug development, especially when many compounds may have comparable pharmacologic properties but differing toxicity profiles (Pallardy et al. 1998). High-throughput assays are also useful for rapid and accurate detection of genetic polymorphisms that could dramatically influence individual differences in drug response (Shi et al. 1999).

Microarrays

Microarray technologies have allowed the development of the field of toxicogenomics, which evaluates changes in genetic response to environmental agents or toxicants. These technologies permit genomewide assessments of changes in gene expression associated with exposure to environmental agents. The identification of responding genes can provide valuable information on cellular response and some information on toxicity pathways that might be affected by environmental agents. Some of the tools and technologies are described below.

Microarrays are high-throughput analytic devices that provide comprehensive genome-scale expression analysis by simultaneously monitoring quantitative transcription of thousands of genes in parallel (Hoheisel 2006). The Affymetrix GeneChip Human Genome U133 Plus 2.0 Array provides comprehensive analysis of genomewide expression of the entire transcribed human genome on a single microarray (Affymetrix Corporation 2007). Whole-genome arrays are also available for the rat and mouse. The use of the rat arrays will probably increase as the relationships between specific genes and markers on the arrays become better understood.

Protein microarrays potentially offer the ability to evaluate all expressed proteins in cells or tissues. Protein-expression profiling would allow some understanding of the relationship between transcription (the suite of mRNAs in the cell) and the translational readout of the transcripts (the proteins). Protein microarrays have diverse applications in biomedical research, including profiling of disease markers and understanding of molecular pathways, protein modifications, and protein activities (Zangar et al. 2005). However, whole-cell or tissue profiling of expressed proteins is still in the developmental stage. These techniques remain expensive, and the technology is in flux.

Differential gene-expression experiments use comparative microarray analysis to identify genes that are upregulated or downregulated in response to experimental conditions. The large-scale investigation of differential gene expression attaches functional activity to structural genomics. Whole-genome-expression experiments involve hundreds of experimental conditions in which patterns of global gene expression are used to classify disease specimens and discover gene functions and toxicogenomic targets (Peeters and Van der Spek 2005). Gene-expression profiling will have a role in identifying toxicity pathways in whole-animal studies but is not expected to be the staple technology for identifying and mapping the pathways.

High-Throughput Functional Genomics[1]

Large-scale evaluations of the status of gene expression and protein concentrations in cells allow understanding of the integrated biologic activities in tissues and can be used to catalog changes after in vivo or in vitro treatment with environmental agents. However, evaluation of the organization and interactions among genes in toxicity pathways requires approaches referred to as functional genomics, which encompass a different suite of molecular tools (Brent 2000). The tools are designed to catalog the full suite of genes that are required for optimal activity of a toxicity pathway. The evaluation of the readout of those functional screens with bioinformatic analysis provides key data about the organization of toxicity pathways and guides computational methods that model the consequences of perturbation of the pathways by environmental agents.

Functional analysis requires a cell-based assay that provides a convenient, automated cell-based measure of functioning of a toxicity pathway (Akutsu et al. 1998; Michiels et al. 2002; Chanda et al. 2003; Lum et al. 2003; Berns et al. 2004; Huang et al. 2004) and requires the ability to automate treatment of the cells with individual cDNAs or small interfering RNAs (siRNAs), which are relatively short RNA oligomers that appear to play important roles in inhibiting gene expression (Hannon 2002; Meister and Tuschl 2004; Mello and Conte 2004; Hammond 2005). Treatment of the cells with a particular cDNA causes overexpression of the gene (and presumably the protein) that is coded by it. In contrast, treatment with gene-specific siRNA causes knockdown of specific proteins by enhancing degradation of the mRNA from the gene.

---

[1]Functional genomics should be distinguished from toxicogenomics. Toxicogenomics is a broad field combining expertise in toxicology, genetics, molecular biology, and environmental health and includes genomics, proteomics, and metabonomics, whereas functional genomics as described here is a specialized discipline that attempts to understand the functions of genes within cellular networks.

High-throughput methods permit automation of such cell-based assays by the use of robots and libraries of cDNAs and siRNAs. The screens show which genes increase and which decrease activity of the toxicity pathway.

Computational Biology

Computational biology uses computer techniques and mathematical modeling to understand biologic processes. It is a powerful tool to cope with the ever-increasing quantity and quality of biologic information on genomics, proteomics, gene expression, gene varieties, genotyping techniques, and protein and cell arrays (Kriete and Eils 2006). Computational tools are used in data analysis, data mining, data integration, network analysis, and multiscale modeling (Kitano 2005). Computational biology is particularly useful for systems biology in understanding structural, regulatory, and kinetic models (Barabasi and Oltvai 2004); in modeling signal transduction (Eungdamrong and Iyengar 2004); and in analyzing genome information and its structural and functional properties (Snitkin et al. 2006). Furthermore, computational biology is used to predict toxic effects of chemical substances (Simon-Hettich et al. 2006), to understand the toxicokinetics and toxicodynamics of xenobiotics (Ekins 2006), to determine gene-expression profiling of cancer cells (Katoh and Katoh 2006), to help in the development of genomic biomarkers (Ginsburg and Haga 2006), and to design virtual experiments to replace or reduce animal testing (Vedani 1999). In drug design and discovery, novel computational technologies help to create chemical libraries of structural motifs relevant to target proteins and their small molecular ligands (Balakin et al. 2006; O'Donoghue et al. 2006).

Cellular signaling circuits handle an enormous variety of functions. Apart from replication and other functions of individual cells, signaling circuits must implement the complex logic of development and function of multicellular organisms. Computer models are helpful in understanding that complexity (Bhalla et al. 2002). Recent studies have extended such models to include electrical, mechanical, and spatial details of signaling (Bhalla 2004a,b). The mitogen-activated protein kinase (MAPK) pathway is one of the most important and extensively studied signaling pathways; it governs growth, proliferation, differentiation, and survival of cells. A wide variety of mathematical models of the MAPK pathway have led to novel insights and predictions as to how it functions (Orton et al. 2005; Santos et al. 2007).

Predictive computational models derived from experimental studies have been developed to describe receptor-mediated cell communication and intracellular signal transduction (Sachs et al. 2005). Physicochemical models attempt to describe biomolecular transformations, such as covalent modification and intermolecular association, with physicochemical equations. The models make specific predictions and work mostly with pathways that are better understood. They can be viewed as translations of familiar pathway maps into mathematical forms (Aldridge et al. 2006). Integrated mechanistic and data-driven modeling for multivariate analysis of signaling pathways is a novel approach to understanding multivariate dependence among molecules in complex networks and potentially can be used to identify combinatorial targets for therapeutic interventions and toxicity-pathway targets that lead to adverse responses (Hua et al. 2006).

In Vivo Tests

As discussed in Chapters 2 and 3, in vivo tests will most likely be used in the foreseeable future to evaluate the formation of metabolites and some mechanistic aspects of target-organ responses to environmental agents, including genomewide evaluation of gene expression. Chapter 3 noted that careful design of those studies could substantially increase the value of information obtained. For example, evaluation of cellular transcriptomic patterns from tissues of animals receiving short-term exposures may provide clues to cellular targets of environmental agents and assist in target-tissue identification. (See Chapter 3 for further discussion of protocol changes that could increase the value of toxicity tests.) Moreover, technologic advances in detection and imaging have the potential for improving in vivo testing. For example, positron-emission tomography (PET) is an imaging tool that can determine biochemical and physiologic processes in vivo by monitoring the activity of radiolabeled compounds (Paans and Vaalburg 2000). Because PET can detect the activity of an administered compound at the cellular level, its use in animal models can result in the incorporation of mechanistic processes and an understanding of the pathologic effects of a candidate compound (Rehmann and Jayson 2005).

TOOLS AND TECHNOLOGIES FOR DOSE-RESPONSE AND EXTRAPOLATION MODELING

As discussed in Chapters 2 and 3, two types of modeling will be critical for implementing the committee's vision: physiologically based pharmacokinetic (PBPK) models and dose-response models of perturbations of toxicity pathways. PBPK models will allow dose extrapolation from in vitro conditions used for assessing toxicity-pathway perturbations to projected human exposures in vivo. Mechanistic models of perturbations of toxicity pathways should aid in developing low-dose extrapolation models that consider the biologic structure of the cellular circuitry controlling pathway activation.

Physiologically Based Pharmacokinetic Models

Assessing the risk associated with human chemical exposure has traditionally relied on the extrapolation of data from animal models to humans, from one route of exposure to another, and from high doses to low doses. Such extrapolation attempts to relate the extent of external exposure to a toxicant to the internal dose in the target tissue of interest. However, differences in biotransformation and other pharmacokinetic processes can introduce error and uncertainty into the extrapolation of toxicity from animals to humans (Kedderis and Lipscomb 2001).

PBPK models provide a physiologic basis for extrapolating between species and routes of exposure and thus allow estimation of the active form of a toxicant that reaches the target tissue after absorption, distribution, and biotransformation (Watanabe et al. 1988). However, PBPK results can differ significantly in the hands of different modelers (Hattis et al. 1990), and improved modeling approaches for parameter selection and uncertainty analysis are under discussion. PBPK models might also be useful for estimating the effect of exposure at different life stages, such as pregnancy, critical periods of development, and childhood growth (Barton 2005). Interindividual differences can be incorporated into PBPK models by integrating quantitative information from in vitro biotransformation studies (Bois et al. 1995; Kedderis and Lipscomb 2001).

The more pervasive use of PBPK approaches in the new strategy for toxicity testing will be in basing dosimetry extrapolations on estimates of partitioning, metabolism, and interactions among chemicals derived from in vitro measurements or perhaps even from SAR or QSAR techniques. Those extrapolations will require some level of validation that might require data from kinetic studies in volunteers or from biomonitoring studies in human populations. In the committee's vision for toxicity testing, the development of PBPK models from SAR predictions of partitioning and metabolism would decrease animal use, and continued improvements in in vitro to in vivo extrapolations of kinetics will support the translation from test-tube studies of perturbations to predictions.

Dose-Response Models of Toxicity Pathways

Dose-response modeling of toxicity pathways involves the integration of mechanistic and dosimetric information about the toxicity of a chemical into descriptive mathematical terms to provide a quantitative model that allows dose and interspecies extrapolation (Conolly 2002). New techniques in molecular biology, such as functional genomics, will play a key role in the development of such models because they provide more detailed information about the organization of toxicity pathways and the dose-response relationships of perturbations of toxicity pathways by environmental agents. Dose-response models have been developed for cell-signaling pathways and used in risk assessment (Andersen et al. 2002). They have found important applications in studying chemical carcinogenesis (Park and Stayner 2006). In particular, models of cancer formation have been developed to describe the induction of squamous-cell carcinomas of the nasal passage in rats exposed to formaldehyde by inhalation, taking into account both tissue dosimetry and the nonlinear effects of cellular proliferation and formation of DNA-protein cross-links (Slikker et al. 2004a, 2004b; Conolly et al. 2004). However, alternative implementations of the formaldehyde model gave substantially different results (Subramaniam et al. 2006). Emerging developments in systems biology allow modeling of cellular and molecular signaling networks affected by chemical exposures and thereby produce an integrated modeling approach capable of predicting dose-response relationships of pathway perturbations by developmental and reproductive toxicants (Andersen et al. 2005b).

In the next decades, the dose-response modeling tools for perturbations should progress relatively rapidly to guide low-dose extrapolations of initial interactions of toxic compounds with biologic systems. The quantitative lineage of early perturbations with apical responses is likely to develop more slowly. For the foreseeable future, the continued refinement of biologic models of signaling circuitry should guide the extrapolation approaches necessary for conducting risk assessment with the toxicity-pathway tests as the cornerstone of toxicity-testing methods.

REFERENCES

Affymetrix Corporation. 2007. GeneChip Arrays. Affymetrix Corporation. [online]. Available: http://www.affymetrix.com/products/arrays/specific/hgu133plus.affx [accessed March 27, 2007].

Akutsu, T., S. Kuhara, O. Maruyama, and S. Miyano. 1998. A system for identifying genetic networks from gene expression patterns produced by gene disruption and overexpressions. Genome Inform. Ser. Workshop Genome Inform. 9:151-160.

Aldridge, B.B., J.M. Burke, D.A. Lauffenburger, and P.K. Sorger. 2006. Physicochemical modeling of cell signaling pathways. Nat. Cell Biol. 8(11):1195-1203.

Andersen, M.E., R.S. Yang, C.T. French, L.S. Chubb, and J.E. Dennison. 2002. Molecular circuits, biological switches, and nonlinear dose-response relationships. Environ. Health Perspect. 110(Suppl. 6):971-978.

Andersen, M.E., J.E. Dennison, R.S. Thomas, and R.B. Conolly. 2005a. New directions in incidence dose-response modeling. Trends Biotechnol. 23(3):122-127.

Andersen, M.E., R.S. Thomas, K.W. Gaido, and R.B. Conolly. 2005b. Dose-response modeling in reproductive toxicology in the systems biology era. Reprod. Toxicol. 19(3):327-337.

Anderson, S. 2002. The state of the world's pharmacy: A portrait of the pharmacy profession. J. Interprof. Care 16(4):391-404.

Balakin, K.V., A.V. Kozintsev, A.S. Kiselyov, and N.P. Savchuk. 2006. Rational design approaches to chemical libraries for hit identification. Curr. Drug Discov. Technol. 3(1):49-65.

Barabasi, A.L., and Z.N. Oltvai. 2004. Network biology: Understanding the cell's functional organization. Nat. Rev. Genet. 5(2):101-113.

Barton, H.A. 2005. Computational pharmacokinetics during developmental windows of susceptibility. J. Toxicol. Environ. Health A 68(11-12):889-900.

Benigni, R. 2004. Chemical structure of mutagens and carcinogens and the relationship with biological activity. J. Exp. Clin. Cancer Res. 23(1):5-8.

Benigni, R., and C. Bossa. 2006. Structure-activity models of chemical carcinogens: State of the art, and new directions. Ann. Ist Super Sanita. 42(2):118-126.

Berns, K., E.M. Hijmans, J. Mullenders, T.R. Brummelkamp, A. Velds, M. Heimerikx, R.M. Kerkhoven, M. Madiredjo, W. Nijkamp, B. Weigelt, R. Agami, W. Ge, G. Cavet, P.S. Linsley, R.L. Beijersbergen, and R. Bernards. 2004. A large-scale RNAi screen in human cells identifies new components of the p53 pathway. Nature 428(6981):431-437.

Bhalla, U.S. 2004a. Signaling in small subcellular volumes. I. Stochastic and diffusion effects on individual pathways. Biophys J. 87(2):733-744.

Bhalla, U.S. 2004b. Signaling in small subcellular volumes. II. Stochastic and diffusion effects on synaptic network properties. Biophys. J. 87(2):745-753.

Bhalla, U.S., P.T. Ram, and R. Iyengar. 2002. MAP kinase phosphatase as a locus of flexibility in a mitogen activated protein kinase signaling network. Science 297(5583):1018-1023.

Bodor, N. 1999. Recent advances in retrometabolic design approaches. J. Control. Release 62(1-2):209-222.

Bois, F.Y., G. Krowech, and L. Zeise. 1995. Modeling human interindividual variability in metabolism and risk: The example of 4-aminobiphenyl. Risk Anal. 15(2):205-213.

Brent, R. 2000. Genomic biology. Cell 100(1):169-183.

Bugrim, A., T. Nikolskaya, and Y. Nikolsky. 2004. Early prediction of drug metabolism and toxicity: Systems biology approach and modeling. Drug Discov. Today 9(3):127-135.

Chanda, S.K., S. White, A.P. Orth, R. Reisdorph, L. Miraglia, R.S. Thomas, P. DeJesus, D.E. Mason, Q. Huang, R. Vega, D.H. Yu, C.G. Nelson, B.M. Smith, R. Terry, A.S. Linford, Y. Yu, G.W. Chirn, C. Song, M.A. Labow, D. Cohen, F.J. King, E.C. Peters, P.G. Schultz, P.K. Vogt, J.B. Hogenesch, and J.S. Caldwell. 2003. Genome-scale functional profiling of the mammalian AP-1signaling pathway. Proc. Natl. Acad. Sci. U.S.A. 100(21):12153-12158.

Congiu, A., D. Pozzi, C. Esposito, C. Castellano, and G. Mossa. 2004. Correlation between structure and transfection efficiency: A study of DC-Chol--DOPE/DNA complexes. Colloids Surf. B Biointerfaces. 36(1):43-48.

Conolly, R.B. 2002. The use of biologically based modeling in risk assessment. Toxicology 27:181-182; 275-279.

Conolly, R.B., J.S. Kimbell, D. Janszen, P.M. Schlosser, D. Kalisak, J. Preston, and F.J. Miller. 2004. Human respiratory tract cancer risks of inhaled formaldehyde: Dose-response predictions derived from biologically-motivated computational modeling of a combined rodent and human dataset. Toxicol. Sci. 82(1):279-296.

Cronin, M.T. 2002. The current status and future applicability of quantitative structure-activity relationships (QSARs) in predicting toxicity. Altern. Lab. Anim. 30(Suppl. 2):81-84.

Cummings, A., and R. Kavlock. 2005. A systems biology approach to developmental toxicology. Reprod. Toxicol. 19(3):281-290.

Daston, G.P. 1997. Advances in understanding mechanisms of toxicity and implications for risk assessment. Reprod. Toxicol. 11(2-3):389-396.

Ekins, S. 2006. Systems-ADME/Tox: Resources and network applications. J. Pharmacol. Toxicol. Methods 53(1):38-66.

Ekins, S., Y. Nikolsky, and T. Nikolskaya. 2005. Techniques: Applications of systems biology to absorption, distribution, metabolism, excretion and toxicity. Trends Pharmacol. Sci. 26(4):202-209.

Eungdamrong, N.J., and R. Iyengar. 2004. Computational approaches for modeling regulatory cellular networks. Trends Cell Biol. 14(12):661-669.

Feher, M., E. Sourial, and J.M. Schmidt. 2000. A simple model for the prediction of blood-brain partitioning. Int. J. Pharm. 201(2):239-247.

Fernandis, A.Z, and M.R. Wenk. 2007. Membrane lipids as signaling molecules. Curr. Opin. Lipidol. 18(2):121-128.

Fischer, H.P. 2005. Towards quantitative biology: Integration of biological information to elucidate disease pathways and to guide drug discovery. Biotechnol. Annu. Rev. 11:1-68.

Ginsburg, G.S., and S.B. Haga. 2006. Translating genomic biomarkers into clinically useful diagnostics. Expert Rev. Mol. Diagn. 6(2):179-191.

Goldberg, A.M., and T. Hartung. 2006. Protecting more than animals. Sci Am. 294(1):84-91.

Gombar, V.K., I.S. Silver, and Z. Zhao. 2003. Role of ADME characteristics in drug discovery and their in silico evaluation: In silico screening of chemicals for their metabolic stability. Curr. Top. Med. Chem. 3(11):1205-1225.

Hammond, S.M. 2005. Dicing and slicing: The core machinery of the RNA interference pathway. FEBS Lett. 579(26):5822-5829.

Hannon, G.J. 2002. RNA interference. Nature 418(6894):244-251.

Hattis, D., P. White, L. Marmorstein, and P. Koch. 1990. Uncertainties in pharmacokinetic modeling for perchloroethylene. I. Comparison of model structure, parameters, and predictions for low-dose metabolism rates for models derived by different authors. Risk Anal. 10(3):449-458.

Hoheisel, J.D. 2006. Microarray technology: Beyond transcript profiling and genotype analysis. Nat. Rev. Genet. 7(3):200-210.

Hua, F., S. Hautaniemi, R. Yokoo, and D.A. Lauffenburger. 2006. Integrated mechanistic and data driven modeling for multivariate analysis of signaling pathways. J. R. Soc. Interface. 3(9):515-526.

Huang, Q., A. Raya, P. DeJesus, S.H. Chao, K.C. Quon, J.S. Caldwell, S.K. Chanda, J.C. Izpisua-Belmonte, and P.G. Schultz. 2004. Identification of p53 regulators by genome-wide functional analysis. Proc. Natl. Acad. Sci. USA 101(10):3456-3461.

Inglese, J. 2002. Expanding the HTS paradigm. Drug Discov. Today 7(Suppl. 18):S105-S106.

Inglese, J., D.S. Auld, A. Jadhav, R.L. Johnson, A. Simeonov, A. Yasgar, W. Zheng, and C.P. Austin. 2006. Quantitative high-throughput screening: A titration-based approach that efficiently identifies biological activities in large chemical libraries. Proc. Natl. Acad. Sci. U.S.A. 103(31):11473-11478.

Katoh, M., and M. Katoh. 2006. Bioinformatics for cancer management in the post-genome era. Technol. Cancer Res. Treat. 5(2):169-175.

Kedderis, G.L, and J.C. Lipscomb. 2001. Application of in vitro biotransformation data and pharmacokinetic modeling to risk assessment. Toxicol. Ind. Health 17(5-10):315-321.

Kitano, H. 2005. International alliance for quantitative modeling in systems biology. Mol. Syst. Biol. 1(1):2005.0007 [online]. Available: http://www.nature.com/msb/journal/v1/n1/pdf/msb4100011.pdf [accessed March 27, 2007]

Kriete, A., and R. Eils. 2006. Introducing computational systems biology. Pp. 1-14 in: Computational System Biology. Boston: Elsevier Academic Press.

Lander, E.S., and R.A. Weinberg. 2000. Genomics: Journey to the center of biology. Science 287(5459):1777-1782.

Lee, M.Y., and J.S. Dordick. 2006. High-throughput human metabolism and toxicity analysis. Curr. Opin. Biotechnol. 17(6):619-627.

Lewin, B., L. Cassimeris, V.R. Lingappa, and G. Plopper. 2007. Cells. Sudbury, MA: Jones and Bartlett Pub.

Lum, L., S. Yao, B. Mozer, A. Rovescalli, D. Von Kessler, M. Nirenberg, and P.A. Beachy. 2003. Identification of Hedgehog pathway components by RNAi in Drosophila cultured cells. Science 299(5615): 2039-2045.

Masimirembwa, C.M., R. Thompson, and T.B. Andersson. 2001. In vitro high throughput screening of compounds for favorable metabolic properties in drug discovery. Comb. Chem. High Throughput Screen. 4(3):245-263.

McKinney, J.D., A. Richard, C. Waller, M.C. Newman, and F. Gerberick. 2000. The practice of structure activity relationships (SAR) in toxicology. Toxicol. Sci. 56(1):8-17.

Meister, G., and T. Tuschl. 2004. Mechanisms of gene slicing by double-stranded RNA. Nature 431(7006):343-349.

Mello, C.C., and D. Conte, Jr. 2004. Revealing the world of RNA interference. Nature 431(7006):338-342.

Michiels, F., H. van Es, L. van Rompaey, P. Merchiers, B. Francken, K. Pittois, J. van der Schueren, R. Brys, J. Vandersmissen, F. Beirinckx, S. Herman, K. Dokic, H. Klaassen, E. Narinx, A. Hagers, W. Laenen, I. Piest, H. Pavliska,

Y. Rombout, E. Langemeijer, L. Ma, C. Schipper, M.D. Raeymaeker, S. Schweicher, M. Jans, K. van Beeck, I.R. Tsang, O. van de Stolpe, P. Tomme, G.J. Arts, and J. Donker. 2002. Arrayed adenoviral expression libraries for functional screening. Nat. Biotechnol. 20(11):1154-1157.

O'Brien, P., and J.R. Haskins. 2007. In vitro cytotoxicity assessment. Methods Mol. Biol. 356: 415-425.

O'Donoghue, S.I., R.B. Russell, and A. Schafferhans. 2006. Three-dimensional structures in target drug discovery and validation. Pp. 285-308 in In Silico Technologies in Drug Target Identification and Validation, 6th Ed, D. Leon, and S. Markel, eds. Boca Raton, FL: CRC Press.

Orton, R.J., O.E. Sturm, V. Vyshemirsky, M. Calder, D.R. Gilbert, and W. Kolch. 2005. Computational modeling of the receptor-tyrosine-kinase-activated MAPK pathway. Biochem. J. 392(Pt. 2):249-261.

Paans, A.M., and W. Vaalburg. 2000. Positron emission tomography in drug development and drug evaluation. Curr. Pharm. Des. 6(16): 1583-1591.

Pallardy, M., S. Kerdine, and H. Lebrec. 1998. Testing strategies in immunotoxicology. Toxicol. Lett. 102-103:257-260.

Park, R.M., and L.T. Stayner. 2006. A search for thresholds and other nonlinearities in the relationship between hexavalent chromium and lung cancer. Risk Anal. 26(1):79-88.

Peeters, J.K., and P.J. Van der Spek. 2005. Growing applications and advancements in microarray technology and analysis tools. Cell Biochem. Biophys. 43(1):149-166.

Potier, M., B. Lakhdar, D. Merlet, and J. Cambar. 1995. Interest and limits of human tissue and cell use in pharmacotoxicology. Cell Biol Toxicol. 11(3-4):133-139.

Rehmann, S., and G.C. Jayson. 2005. Molecular imaging of antiangiogenic agents. Oncologist. 10(2):92-103.

Sachs, K., O. Perez, D. Pe'er, D.A. Lauffenburger, and G.P. Nolan. 2005. Causal protein-signaling networks derived from multiparameter single-cell data. Science 308(5721):523-529.

Santos, S.D., P.J. Verveer, and P.I. Bastiaens. 2007. Growth factor-induced MAPK network topology shapes Erk response determining PC-12 cell fate. Nat. Cell Biol. 9(3):324-330.

Schleger, C., S.J. Platz, and U. Deschl. 2004. Development of an in vitro model for vascular injury with human endothelial cells. ALTEX 21(Suppl. 3):12-19.

Schultz, T.W., and J.R. Seward. 2000. Health effects related structure-toxicity relationships: A paradigm for the first decade of the new millennium. Sci. Total Environ. 249(1-3):73-84.

Schultz, T.W., G.D. Sinks, and A.P. Bearden. 1998. QSAR in aquatic toxicology: A mechanism of action approach comparing toxic potency to *Pimephales pro-*

melas, Tetrahymena pyriformis, and *Vibrio fischeri.* Pp. 51-110 in Comparative QSAR, J. Devillers, ed. London: Taylor and Francis.

Shi, M.M., M.R. Bleavins, and F.A. de la Iglesia. 1999. Technologies for detecting genetic polymorphisms in pharmacogenomics. Mol. Diagn. 4(4):343-351.

Simon-Hettich, B., A. Rothfuss, and T. Steger-Hartmann. 2006. Use of computer-assisted prediction of toxic effects of chemical substances. Toxicology 224(1-2):156-162.

Slikker, W., Jr., M.E. Andersen, M.S. Bogdanffy, J.S. Bus, S.D. Cohen, R.B. Conolly, R.M. David, N.G. Doerrer, D.C. Dorman, D.W. Gaylor, D. Hattis, J.M. Rogers, R.W. Setzer, J.A. Swenberg, and K. Wallace. 2004a. Dose-dependent transitions in mechanisms of toxicity: Case studies. Toxicol. Appl. Pharmacol. 201(3):226-294.

Slikker, W., Jr., M.E. Andersen, M.S. Bogdanffy, J.S. Bus, S.D. Cohen, R.B. Conolly, R.M. David, N.G. Doerrer, D.C. Dorman, D.W. Gaylor, D. Hattis, J.M. Rogers, R. Woodrow Setzer, J.A. Swenberg, and K. Wallace. 2004b. Dose-dependent transitions in mechanisms of toxicity. Toxicol. Appl. Pharmacol. 201(3):203-225.

Slikker, W., Z. Xu, and C. Wang. 2005. Application of a systems biology approach to developmental neurotoxicology. Reprod. Toxicol. 19(3):305-319.

Snitkin, E.S., A.M. Gustafson, J. Mellor, J. Wu, and C. DeLisi. 2006. Comparative assessment of performance and genome dependence among phylogenetic profiling methods. BMC Bioinformatics 7:420.

Soffers, A.E., M.G. Boersma, W.H. Vaes, J. Vervoort, B. Tyrakowska, J.L. Hermens, I.M. Rietjens. 2001. Computer-modeling-based QSARs for analyzing experimental data on biotransformation and toxicity. Toxicol. In Vitro 15(4-5):539-551.

Spielmann, H., and M. Liebsch. 2001. Lessons learned from validation of in vitro toxicity test: From failure to acceptance into regulatory practice. Toxicol. In Vitro 15(4-5):585-590.

Subramaniam, R.P., K.S. Crump, C. Chen, P. White, C. Van Landingham, J.F. Fox, P. Schlosser, T.R. Covington, D. DeVoney, J.J. Vandenberg, P. Preuss, and J. Whalan. 2006. The role of mutagenicity in describing formaldehyde-induced carcinogenicity: Possible inferences using the ciit model. Presented at the Society of Risk Analysis Annual Meeting, Dec. 3-6, 2006, Baltimore, MD.

Suemori, H. 2006. Establishment and therapeutic use of human embryonic stem cell lines. Hum. Cell. 19(2):65-70.

Suzuki, N., A. Higashiguchi, Y. Hasegawa, H. Matsumoto, S. Oie, K. Orikawa, S. Ezawa, N. Susumu, K. Miyashita, and D. Aoki. 2005. Loss of integrin alpha3 expression is associated with acquisition of invasive potential by ovarian clear cell adenocarcinoma cells. Hum. Cell. 8(3):147-155.

Tong, W., W.J. Welsh, L. Shi, H. Fang, and R. Perkins. 2003. Structure-activity relationship approaches and applications. Environ. Toxicol. Chem. 22(8): 1680-1695.

van den Broek, L.A., E. Lazaro, Z. Zylicz, P.J. Fennis, F.A. Missler, P. Lelieveld, M. Garzotto, D.J. Wagener, J.P. Ballesta, and H.C. Ottenheijm. 1989. Lipophilic analogues of sparsomycin as strong inhibitors of protein synthesis and tumor growth: A structure-activity relationship study. J. Med. Chem. 32(8):2002-2015.

Van der Berg, M., L. Birnbaum, A.T. Bosveld, B. Brunstrom, P. Cook, M. Feeley, J.P. Giesy, A. Hanberg, R. Hasegawa, S.W. Kennedy, T. Kubiak, J.C. Larsen, F.X. van Leeuwen, A.K. Liem, C. Nolt, R.E. Peterson, L. Poellinger, S. Safe, D. Schrenk, D. Tillitt, M. Tysklind, M. Younes, F. Waern, and T. Zacharewski. 1998. Toxic equivalency factors (TEFs) for PCBs, PCDDs, PCDFs for human and wildlife. Environ. Health Perspect. 106(12):775-792.

Vedani, A. 1999. Replacing animal testing by virtual experiments: A challenge in computational biology. Chimia 53(5):227-228.

Walker, J.D., M. Enache, and J.C. Dearden. 2003a. Quantitative cationic-activity relationships for predicting toxicity of metals. Environ. Toxicol. Chem. 22(8):1916-1935.

Walker, J.D., J. Jaworska, M.H. Comber, T.W. Schultz, and J.C. Dearden. 2003b. Guidelines for developing and using quantitative structure-activity relationships. Environ. Toxicol. Chem. 22(8):1653-1665.

Walker, J.D., ed. 2004. Quantitative Structure–Activity Relationships for Pollution Prevention, Toxicity Screening, Risk Assessment, and Web Applications (QSAR II). Pensacola, FL: SETAC Press.

Wang, S.L., F.H. Lan, Y.P. Zhuang, H.Z. Li, L.H. Huang, D.Z. Zheng, J. Zeng, L.H. Dong, Z.Y. Zhu, and J.L. Fu. 2006. Microarray analysis of gene-expression profile in hepatocellular carcinoma cell, BEL-7402, with stable suppression of hLRH-1 via a DNA vector-based RNA interference. Yi Chuan Xue Bao. 33(10):881-891.

Waring, J.F., and R.G. Ulrich. 2000. The impact of genomics based technologies on drug safety evaluation. Annu. Rev. Pharmacol. Toxicol. 40:335-352.

Watanabe, P.G., A.M. Schumann, and R.H. Reitz. 1988. Toxicokinetics in the evaluation of toxicity data. Regul. Toxicol. Pharmacol. 8(4):408-413.

Zangar, R.C., S.M. Varnum, and N. Bollinger. 2005. Studying cellular processes and detecting disease with protein microarrays. Drug Metab. Rev. 37(3): 473-487.

5

Developing the Science Base
and Assays to Implement the Vision

Rapid advances in the understanding of the organization and function of biologic systems provide the opportunity to develop innovative mechanistic approaches to toxicity testing. In comparison with the current system, the new approaches should provide wider coverage of chemicals of concern, reduce the time needed for generating toxicity-test data required for decision-making, and use animals to a far smaller extent. Accordingly, the committee has proposed development of a testing structure that evaluates perturbations in toxicity pathways and relies on a mix of high- and medium-throughput assays and targeted in vivo tests as the foundation of its vision for toxicity testing. This chapter discusses the kinds of applied and basic research needed to support the new toxicity-testing approach, the institutional resources required to support and encourage it, and the valuable products that can be expected during the transition from the current apical end-point testing to a mechanistically based in vivo and in vitro test system.

Most tests in the committee's vision would be unlike current toxicity tests, which generate data on apical end points. The mix of tests in the vision include in vitro tests that assess critical mechanistic end points involved in the induction of overt toxic effects rather than the effects themselves and targeted in vivo tests that ensure adequate testing of metabolites and coverage of end points. The move toward a mechanism-oriented testing paradigm poses challenges. Implementation will require (1) the availability of suites of in vitro tests—preferably based on human cells, cell lines, or components—that are sufficiently comprehensive to evaluate activity in toxicity pathways associated with the broad array of possible toxic responses; (2) the availability of targeted tests to complement the in vitro tests and ensure overall adequate data for decision-making; (3) models of toxicity pathways to support application of in vitro test results to predict general-population exposures that could potentially cause adverse perturbations; (4) infrastructure changes to support the basic and applied research needed to develop the tests and the pathway models; (5) validation of tests and test strategies for incorporation into chemical-assessment guidelines that will provide direction on interpreting and drawing conclusions from the new assay results; and (6) acceptance of the idea that the results of tests based on perturbations in toxicity pathways are adequately predictive of adverse responses and can be used in decision-making. Development of the new assays and the related basic research—the focus of this chapter—requires a substantial research investment over quite a few years. Institutional acceptance of the new tests and the requisite new risk-assessment approaches—the focus of Chapter 6—also require careful planning. They cannot occur overnight.

Ultimately, the time required to conduct the research needed to support large-scale incorporation of the new mechanistic assays into a test strategy that can adequately and rapidly address large numbers of agents depends on the institutional will to commit resources to support the changes. The committee believes that with a concerted research effort, over the next 10 years high-throughput test batteries could be developed that would substantially improve the ability to identify toxicity hazards caused by a number of mechanisms of action. Those results in themselves would be a considerable advance. The time for full realization of the new test strategy, with its mix of in vitro and in vivo test batteries that can rapidly and inexpensively assess large numbers of substances with adequate coverage of possible end points, could be 20 or more years.

This chapter starts by discussing basic research that will provide the foundation for assay development. It then outlines a research strategy and milestones. It concludes by discussing the scientific infrastructure that will support the basic and applied research required to develop the high-throughput and targeted testing strategy envisioned by the committee.

SCOPE OF SCIENTIFIC KNOWLEDGE, METHODS, AND ASSAY DEVELOPMENT

This section outlines the scientific inquiry required to develop the efficient and effective testing strategy envisioned by the committee. Several basic-research questions need to be addressed to develop the knowledge base from which toxicity-pathway assays and supporting testing technologies can be designed. The discussion here is intended to provide a broad overview, not a detailed research agenda. The committee recognizes the challenges and effort involved in addressing some of these research questions.

Knowledge Development

Knowledge critical for the development of high-throughput assays is emerging from biologic, medical, and pharmaceutical research. Further complementary, focused research will be needed to address fully the key questions that when answered will support toxicity-pathway assay development. Those questions are outlined in Box 5-1 and elaborated below.

• *Toxicity-pathway identification.* The key pathways that, when sufficiently perturbed, will result in toxicity will be identified primarily from future, current, and completed studies in the basic biology of cell-signaling motifs. Identification will involve the discovery of the protein components of toxicity pathways and how the pathways are altered by environmental agents. Many pathways are under investigation with respect to the basic biology of cellular processes. For example, the National Institutes of Health (NIH) has a major program under way to develop high-throughput screening (HTS) assays based on important biologic responses in in vitro systems. HTS has the potential to identify chemical probes of genes, pathways, and cell functions that may ultimately lead to characterization of the relationship between chemical structure and biologic activity (Inglese et al. 2006). Determining the number and nature of toxicity pathways involved in human disease and impairment is an essential component of the committee's vision for toxicity testing.

• *Multiple pathways.* Adverse biologic change can occur from simultaneous perturbations of multiple toxicity pathways. Environmental agents typically affect more than one toxicity pathway. Although the committee envisions the design of a suite of toxicity tests that will provide broad coverage of biologic perturbations in all key toxicity pathways, biologic perturbations in different pathways may lead to synergistic interactions with important implications for human health. For some adverse health effects, an understanding of the interplay of multiple pathways involved may be important. For others, the research need will be to identify the pathway affected at the lowest dose of the environmental agent.

BOX 5-1 Key Research Questions in Developing Knowledge
to Support Pathway Testing

Toxicity-Pathway Identification—What are the key pathways whose
   perturbations result in toxicity?
Multiple Pathways—What alteration in response can be expected from
   simultaneous perturbations of multiple toxicity pathways?
Adversity—What adverse effects are linked to specific toxicity-pathway
   perturbations? What patterns and magnitudes of perturbations
   are predictive of adverse health outcomes?
Life Stages—How can the perturbations of toxicity pathways associated
   with developmental timing or aging be best captured to enable
   the advancement of high-throughput assays?
Effects of Exposure Duration—How are biologic responses affected by
   exposures of different duration?
Low-Dose Response—What is the effect on a toxicity pathway of adding
   small amounts of toxicants in light of pre-existing endogenous
   and exogenous human exposures?
Human Variability—How do people differ in their expression of toxicity-
   pathway constituents and in their predisposition to disease and
   impairment?

- *Adversity.* An understanding of possible diseases or functional losses that may result from specific toxicity-pathway perturbations will support the use of pathway perturbations for decision-making. Current risk assessments rely on toxicity tests that
demonstrate apical adverse health effects, such as disease or functional deficits, that are at various distances downstream of the toxicity-pathway perturbations. In the committee's vision, the assessment of potential human health impact will be based on
perturbations in toxicity pathways. For example, activation of estrogenic action to abnormal levels during pregnancy is associated
with undescended testes and, in later life, testicular cancer. Research will be needed to understand the patterns and magnitudes
of the perturbations that will lead to adverse effects. As part of the

research, biomarkers of effect that can be monitored in humans and studied in whole animals will be useful.

- *Life stages.* An understanding of how pathways associated with developmental timing or aging can be adversely perturbed and lead to toxicity will be needed to develop high-throughput assays that can capture and adequately cover developmental and senescing life stages. Many biologic functions require coordination and integration of a wide array of cellular signals that interact through broad networks that contribute to biologic function at different life stages. That complexity of pathway interaction holds for reproductive and developmental functions, which are governed by parallel and sequential signaling networks during critical periods of biologic development. Because of the complexity of such pathways, the challenge will be to identify all important pathways that affect such functions to ensure adequate protection against risks to the fetus and infant. That research will involve elucidating temporal changes in key toxicity pathways that might occur during development and the time-dependent effects of exposure on these pathways.

- *Effects of exposure duration.* The dose of and response to exposure to a toxicant in the whole organism depend on the duration of exposure. Thus, conventional toxicity testing places considerable emphasis on characterizing risks associated with exposures of different duration, from a few days to the test animal's lifetime. The ultimate goal in the new paradigm is to evaluate conditions under which human cells are likely to respond and to ensure that these conditions do not occur in exposures of human populations. Research will be needed to understand how the dose-response relationships for perturbations might change with the duration of exposure and to understand pathway activation under acute, subchronic, and chronic exposure conditions. The research will involve investigating the differential responses of cells of various ages and backgrounds to a toxic compound and possible differences in responses of cells between people of different ages.

• *Low-dose response.* The assessment of the potential for an adverse health effect from a small environmental exposure involves an understanding of how the small exposure adds to pre-existing exposures that affect the same toxicity pathways and disease processes. For the more common human diseases and impairments, a myriad of exposures from food, pharmaceuticals, the environment, and endogenous processes have the potential to perturb underlying toxicity pathways. Understanding how a specific environmental exposure contributes, with the other exposures, to modulate a toxicity pathway is critical for the understanding of low-dose response. Because the toxicity tests used in the committee's long-range vision are based largely on cellular assays involving sensitive biomarkers of alterations in biologic function, it will be possible to study the potential for adverse human health effects at doses lower than is possible with conventional whole-animal tests. Given the cost-effectiveness of the computational methods and in vitro tests that form the core of the toxicity testing, it will be efficient to evaluate effects at multiple doses and so build a basis of detailed dose-response research.

• *Human variability.* People differ in their expression of toxicity-pathway constituents and consequently in their predisposition to disease and impairment. An understanding of differences among people in the level of responsiveness of particular toxicity pathways is needed to interpret the importance of small environmental exposures. The comprehensive mapping of toxicity pathways provides an unprecedented opportunity to identify gene loci and other determinants of human sensitivity to environmental exposures. That research will support the development of biomarkers of exposure, effect, and susceptibility for surveillance in the human population, and these discoveries in turn will support an assessment of host susceptibility for use in extrapolating results from the in vitro assays to the general population and susceptible groups. The enhanced ability to characterize interindividual differences in sensitivity to environmental exposures will provide a firmer scientific basis of the establishment of human exposure guidelines that can protect susceptible subpopulations.

Research on most, or all, of the above subjects is going on in the United States and internationally. It is taking place in academe, industry, and government institutions and is funded by foundations and the federal government mainly to understand the basis of human disease and treatment. Private firms, such as pharmaceutical and biotechnology companies, conduct the research for product development. However, efforts directed specifically toward developing toxicity-testing systems are small.

Test and Analytic Methods Development

The research described above will provide the foundation for the development of toxicity tests and comprehensive testing approaches. The categories of toxicity tests and methods to be developed are outlined below, and the primary questions to be answered in their development are presented in Box 5-2.

• *Methods to predict metabolism.* A key issue to address at an early phase will be development of methods to ensure adequate testing for metabolites in high-throughput assays. Understanding the range of metabolic products and the variation in metabolism among humans and being able to simulate human metabolism as needed in test systems are critical for developing valid toxicity-pathway assays. Without such methods, targeted in vivo assays will be needed to evaluate metabolism.

• *Chemical-characterization tools.* In addition to metabolism, further development of tools to support chemical characterization

---

BOX 5-2 Main Questions in Developing Tests and Methods

Methods to Predict Metabolism—How can adequate testing for
  metabolites in the high-throughput assays be ensured?
Chemical-Characterization Tools—What computational tools can best
  predict chemical properties, metabolites, xenobiotic-cellular and
  molecular interactions, and biologic activity?
Assays to Uncover Cell Circuitry—What methods will best facilitate the
  discovery of the circuitry associated with toxicity pathways?
Assays for Large-Scale Application—Which assays best capture the
  elucidated pathways and best reflect in vivo conditions? What
  designs will ensure adequate testing of volatile compounds?
Suite of Assays—What mix of pathway-based high- and medium-
  throughput assays and targeted tests will provide adequate
  coverage? What targeted tests should be developed to complement
  the toxicity-pathway assays? What are the appropriate positive and
  negative controls that should be used to validate the assay suite?
Human-Surveillance Strategy—What surveillance is needed to interpret
  the results of pathway tests in light of variable human
  susceptibility and background exposures?
Mathematical Models for Data Interpretation and Extrapolation—What
  procedures should be used to evaluate whether humans are at risk
  from environmental exposures?
Test-Strategy Uncertainty—How can the overall uncertainty in the
  testing strategy be best evaluated?

---

will be important. The tools will include computational and structure-activity relationship (SAR) methods to predict chemical
properties, potential initial interactions of a chemical and its metabolites with cellular molecules, and biologic activity. A National
Research Council report (NRC 2000) indicated that early cellular
interactions are important in understanding potential toxicity and
include receptor-ligand interactions, covalent binding with DNA
and other endogenous molecules, peroxidation of lipids and proteins, interference with sulfhydryl groups, DNA methylation, and

o

inhibition of protein function. Good predictive methods for chemical characterization will reduce the need for targeted testing and enhance the efficiency of the testing.

• *Assays to uncover cell circuitry.* Development of methods to facilitate the discovery of the circuitry associated with toxicity pathways will involve functional genomic techniques for integrating and interpreting various data types and for translating dose-response relationships from simple to complex biologic systems, for example, from the pathway to the tissue level. It will most likely require improved methods in bioinformatics, systems biology, and computational toxicology. Some advances in overexpression with complementary DNA (cDNA) and gene knockdown with small inhibitory RNAs are likely to allow improved pathway mapping and will also lead to studies with cells or cell lines that are more readily transfectable.

• *Assays for large-scale application.* Several substantive issues will need to be considered in developing assays for routine application in a testing strategy. First, as pathways are identified, medium- and high-throughput assays that adequately evaluate pathways and human biology will be developed, including new, preferably human, cell-based cultures for assessment of perturbations. Second, the assay designs that best capture the elucidated pathways and can be applied for rapid large-scale testing of chemicals will need to be identified. Third, an important design criterion for assays will be that they are adequately reflective of the in vivo cellular environment. For any given assay, that will involve an understanding of the elements of the human cellular environment that must be simulated and of culture conditions that affect response. Fourth, the molecular evolution of cell lines during passage in culture and related interlaboratory differences that can result will have to be controlled for. Fifth, approaches for the testing of volatile compounds will require early attention in the development of high-throughput assays; this has been a challenge for in vitro test systems in general. Sixth, assay sensitivity (the probability that the assay identifies the phenomenon that it is designed to identify) and assay specificity (the probability that the assay does not identify a phenomenon as occurring when it does not) will be important considerations in assay design. Individual assays and test batteries should have the capability to predict accurately the effects that they are designed to measure without undue numbers of false positives and false negatives. And seventh, it will be important to achieve flexibility to expand or contract the suites of assays as more detailed biologic understanding of health and disease states emerges from basic research studies.

• *Suite of assays.* An important criterion for the development of a suite of assays for assessing the potential for a substance to cause a particular type of disease or group of toxicities will be adequate coverage of causative mechanisms, affected cell types, and susceptible individuals. Ensuring the right mix of pathway-based high-throughput assays and targeted tests will involve research. For diseases for which toxicity pathways are not fully understood, targeted in vivo or other tests may be included to ensure adequate coverage.

• *Human-surveillance strategy.* Human data on the fundamental biologic events involved in the activation of toxicity pathways will aid the interpretation of the results of high-throughput assays. They will provide the basis of understanding of determinants of human susceptibilities related to a toxicity pathway and of background exposures to compounds affecting the pathway. Research will be needed to assess how population-based studies can best be designed and conducted to complement high-throughput testing and provide the information necessary for data interpretation.

• *Mathematical models for data interpretation and extrapolation.* Procedures for evaluating the impact of human exposure concentrations will involve pharmacokinetic and other modeling methods to relate cell media concentrations to human tissue doses and biomonitoring data and to account for exposure patterns and interindividual variabilities. To facilitate interpretation of high-throughput assay results, models of toxicity pathways (see Chapter 3) and other techniques will be needed to address differences among people in their levels of activation of particular response pathways. Although it is not a key aspect of the current vision, in the distant future research may enable the development of biologically based dose-response models of apical responses for risk prediction.

• *Test-strategy uncertainty.* Methods to evaluate the overall uncertainty in a possible testing strategy will assist the validation and evolution of the new methods. Formal methods could be developed that use systematic approaches to evaluate uncertainty in predicting from the test battery results the doses that should be without biologic effect in human populations. These uncertainty evaluations can be used in the construction and selection of testing strategies.

Whether the testing strategy will detect and predict harmful exposures will depend on whether the major toxicity pathways are addressed by the high-throughput assays or covered by the targeted in vivo and other tests. To ensure that the test system is adequate, the committee envisions a multipronged approach that includes the following components:

• A continuing research and evaluation program to develop, improve, and assess the testing program.

• Adequate validation of the assays, including examination of false-negative and false-positive rates, by applying the assays to sufficient numbers of chemicals of known toxicity.

• A robust program of biomonitoring, human health surveillance, and molecular epidemiology to assess exposures and early indicators of toxicity, to aid in interpretation of high-throughput assay results, and to monitor exposures to ensure that toxic ones are not missed.

Aspects of those endeavors are discussed in the following sections.

STRATEGY FOR KNOWLEDGE AND ASSAY DEVELOPMENT AND VALIDATION

The research strategy to develop the computational tools, suites of in vitro assays, and complementary targeted tests envisioned by the committee will likely involve contributions on multiple fronts, including the following:

• Basic biologic research to obtain the requisite knowledge of toxicity pathways and the potential human health impacts when the pathways are perturbed.
• Science and technology milestones that ensure timely achievement of assays and tool development for the new paradigm.
• Phased basic and applied research to demonstrate success in the transition to the testing emphasis on toxicity pathways.

The basic-research effort will be directed at discovering and mapping toxicity pathways that are the early targets of perturbation by environmental agents and at understanding how agents cause the perturbations. That will be followed by research focused on the design of assays that can be used to determine, first, whether an agent has the potential to perturb the pathway and, if so, the levels and durations of exposure required. The scientific inquiry will involve research at multiple levels of biologic organization, that is, understanding the nature of toxicity pathways at the molecular and cellular levels and how toxicity-pathway alterations may translate to disease processes in tissues, organs, and the whole organism. Some of the tools and technologies that enable this research are described in Chapter 4.

In each broad field of toxicity testing, such as neurotoxicology and reproductive and developmental toxicity, systematic approaches to assay development, assay validation, and generalized acceptance of the assays will be organized and pursued. As the research questions presented in the previous section are answered, milestones would be achieved in an orderly manner. Some important milestones to move from pathway research through assay development to validated test strategies are presented in broad brush strokes in Box 5-3. The committee recognizes that the implementation of its recommendations would entail extensive planning and expert deliberation; through those processes, the important milestones would be subdivided, elaborated, reshaped, and perhaps even replaced.

The research would progress in sequential phases, whose timelines would overlap. The committee finds that four phases would evolve as follows:

Phase I: Toxicity-pathway elucidation. A focused research effort is pursued first to understand the toxicity pathways for a select group of health effects (that is, apical end points) or molecular mechanisms. Early in this first phase, a data-storage, -access, and -management system would be established to enable broad use of the data being generated to facilitate the understanding of the toxicity pathways and research and knowledge development in later phases. A third element of this phase would involve developing standard practices for research methods and reporting of results so that they are understandable and accessible to a broad audience of researchers and to facilitate consistency and validity in the research methods used. Research in this phase would also focus on developing tools for predicting metabolism, characterizing chemicals, and planning a strategy for human surveillance and biomonitoring of exposure, susceptibility, and effect markers associated with the toxicity-pathway perturbations.

BOX 5-3 Some Science and Technology Milestones in Developing Toxicity-Pathway Tests As the Cornerstone of Future Toxicity-Testing Strategies

Develop rapid methods and systems to enable in vitro dosing with chemical stressors (including important metabolites and volatile compounds).
Create and adapt human, human-gene-transfected rodent, and other cell lines and systems, with culture medium conditions, to have an adequate array of in vitro human cell and tissue surrogates.
Adapt and develop technologies to enable the full elucidation of critical toxicity pathways causing the diseases by the mechanisms selected for pilot project study.
Develop toxicity-pathway assays that fully explore the possible effects of exogenous chemical exposure on the diseases and mechanisms selected for a pilot-project study, thereby demonstrating proof of concept.
Establish efficient approaches for validating suites of high-throughput assays.
Develop the infrastructure for data management, assay standardization, and reporting to enable broad data-sharing across academic, government, industry, and nongovernment-organization sectors and institutions.

Phase II: Assay development and validation. High- and medium-throughput assays would be developed for toxicity pathways and points for chemical perturbation in the pathways organized for assay development. During this phase, attempts would be pursued to develop biologic markers of exposure, susceptibility, and effect for use in surveillance and biomonitoring of human populations where these toxicity pathways might activated.

Phase III: Assay relevance and validity trial. The third phase would explore assay use, usually in parallel with traditional apical tests. It would screen chemicals that would not otherwise be tested and would begin the biomonitoring and surveillance of human populations.

Phase IV: Assembly and validation of test batteries. Suites of assays would be proposed and validated for use in place of identified apical tests.

Some of the key science and technology development activities for the phases are listed out in Figure 5-1, and some of the critical aspects are described below. All phases would include research on toxicity pathways. Progression through the phases would involve exploring the research questions outlined in Box 5-1.

Phase I: Toxicity-Pathway Elucidation

Research to Understand Toxicity Pathways

Phase I research would develop pathway knowledge from which assays for health effects would emerge. Systems-biology approaches—including molecular profiling microarrays, pathway mining, and other high-resolution techniques—would reveal key molecular interactions. Mechanistic understanding provides the basis for identifying the key molecular "triggers" or mechanisms of interactions that can alter biologic processes and ultimately cause toxicity after an environmental exposure. Those nodal triggers or interactions would be modeled in vitro and computationally to provide a suite of appropriate assays for detecting toxicity-pathway perturbations and the requisite tools for describing dose-response relationships.

Early efforts would explore possible toxicity pathways for health effects where there is fairly advanced knowledge of mechanisms of toxicity, molecular signaling and interactions. As a

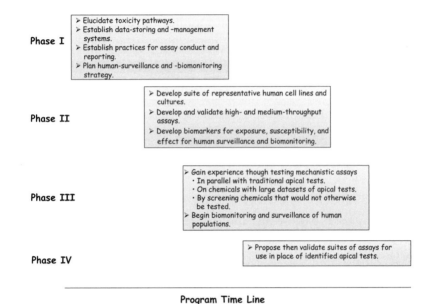

Program Time Line

FIGURE 5-1 Progression of some important science and technology activities during assay development.

case study, the following sketches out how knowledge development might begin for toxic responses that are associated with estrogenic signaling alterations caused by agonists and antagonists of estrogen function.

Even our current appreciation of the number of potential toxicity pathways highlights the breadth of responses that might be evaluated in various high-throughput assays. Consideration of adverse responses at the level of the intact organism that might be associated with altered signaling through estrogen-receptor-mediated responses illustrates some of the challenges. Xenobiotic-caused alteration in estrogen signaling can occur or be measured at a number of points in the various process that affect estrogen actions, including steroidogenesis, hormone transport and elimination, receptor binding and alteration in numbers of receptors, and changes in nuclear translocation. Those pathways may also be evaluated at different levels of organization—ligand binding, receptor translocation, transcriptional activation, and integrated cellular responses. Some of the processes are outlined here.

- *Estrogen steroidogenesis.* Upstream alterations in steroidogenesis pathways or other independently regulated pathways that affect endocrine signaling would be explored. Knowledge development would focus on understanding of enzymatic function for key steroidogenesis pathways and the interactions of the pathways with each other and on understanding of how key elements of the pathways might be altered, including alterations of precursors, products, and metabolites when pathway dysregulation occurs. The research might involve quantitative assessment of key enzyme functions in in vitro and in vivo systems, analytic techniques to measure various metabolites, and modeling to understand the target and key steps that undergo estrogen-related dysregulation. Other assays would develop SAR information on compounds already associated with altered steroidogenesis in other situations.

- *Estrogen-receptor interactions.* Much is known about the molecular interactions between xenobiotics and estrogen receptors (ERs), for example, direct xenobiotic interaction with ERs, including differential interaction with specific ER subtypes, such as ER-α and ER-β xenobiotic interactions with discrete receptor domains that give rise to different biologic consequences, such as interactions with the ligand-binding domain that could cause conformational changes that activate or inhibit signaling; and direct xenobiotic interactions with other components of the ER complex, including accessory proteins, coactivators, and other coregulatory elements. Most responses associated with altered estrogen signaling would be more easily evaluated in assays that evaluated a larger-scale function, such as receptor activation of estrogen-mediated transcription of reporter genes or estrogen-mediated cell responses (for example, cell proliferation of estrogen-sensitive cells in vitro).

- *Processes that lead to estrogenic transgenerational epigenetic effects.* Assay development to address estrogen-induced transgenerational epigenetic effects would involve understanding how early-life exposures to estrogenic compounds permanently alter transcriptional control of genes, understanding how such early-life exposures might be priming events for later-life alterations in reproductive competence or the development of cancer, and understanding how such exposures may produce transgenerational effects. Specific approaches in this research might include genomewide methods to analyze the patterns of DNA methylation with and without estrogenic exposure, quantification of histone modifications, measurements of microRNAs, and the dissection and mechanistic understanding of hormonal inputs to the epigenetic regulatory phenomena.

Those are just a few examples of the kinds of research on estrogenic compounds that would support assay development. The approaches include relatively small-scale research efforts for processes that are fairly well understood (such as direct ligand-receptor interactions) and larger endeavors for the yet-to-be-explained (such as the epigenetic and transgenerational effects of early-life estrogenic-compound exposure). A holistic understanding of estrogenic and other pathways and signaling in humans would be derived incrementally by building on studies in a wide variety of species and tissues. New information from basic studies in biology is likely to lead to improved assays for testing specific toxicity pathways.

The identified estrogenic pathways and signaling processes, once understood, would serve as the substrate for further pathway mining to highlight the critical events that could be tested experimentally in assay systems, that is, events that are obligatory for downstream, apical responses and occur at the lowest exposure of a biologic system to an environmental agent. With studies on the organization of response circuitry controlling the toxicity-pathway responses, a dose-response model would be based on key, nodal points in the circuits that control perturbations rather than on the overall detail of all steps in the signaling process.

Assessing Validity of Pathway Knowledge and Linkage to Adversity at the Organism Level

The next step in pathway elucidation would be the assessment of the validity of the pathway knowledge, which would proceed in two steps and involve the broader scientific community.

First, the validity would be tested by artificially modulating the pathways to establish that predicted downstream molecular consequences are consistent and measurable. The perturbations could take place, for example, with the use of standard reference compounds, such as 17β-estradiol, or discrete molecular probes, such as genetically modified test systems, knockout models, or other interventions with siRNA or small-molecule inhibitors of key enzymes of other cellular factors.

Second, the consequences of pathway disruption for the organism—the linkage of molecular events to downstream established biologic effects considered to be adverse or human disease—would be assessed. For the case of perturbations of estrogen signaling, it may include linkage with results from short-term in vivo assays, such as an increase in uterine weight in rats in the uterotrophic assay. The link between the toxicity pathways and adverse effects at the level of the whole organism would be assessed in a variety of in vivo and in vitro experiments.

Development of Data-Storage, Data-Access, and Data-Management Systems

Very early stage in Phase I, data-storage, -access, and -management systems should be developed and standardized. As the altered-estrogen-signaling case study indicates, the acquisition of the knowledge to develop high-throughput testing assays would involve the discovery of toxicity pathways and networks from vast amounts of data from studies of biologic circuitry and interactions of environmental agents with the circuitry. Organization of that knowledge would require data analysis and exploration by interdisciplinary teams of scientists. Understanding the relationships of pathways to adverse end points would also involve large-volume data analysis, as would the design of test batteries and their validation. Those efforts could be stymied without easy and wide public access to databases of results from a broad array of research studies: high-throughput assays, quantitative-SAR model development, protein and DNA microarrays, pharmacokinetic and metabolomic experiments, in vivo apical tests, and human biomonitoring, clinical, and population-based studies. Central repositories for -omics data are under development and exist to a small extent for some in vivo toxicity data. The scale of data storage and access envisioned by the committee is much larger.

The data should be available, regardless of whether they were generated by industry, academe, federal institutions, or foundations. However, the data-management system must also be able to accommodate confidential data but allow for data-sharing of confidential components of the database among parties that agree to the terms of confidentiality. The data-management system would also provide procedures and guidelines for adequate quality control. Central storage efforts would need to be coordinated and standardized as appropriate to ensure usefulness.

Standardization of Research Assays and Results

With the development of data-management systems, processes for standardizing platforms would have to be developed. Currently, there is little standardization of microarrays, although such efforts are moving more quickly with the Minimum Information About a Microarray Experiment formats now in use (Brazma et al. 2001). Too much standardization can stifle innovation, so approaches to identifying and using the appropriate level of standardization would be needed. Bioinformatics should proceed jointly with the development of assay-platform technology. Data-management systems would have to evolve flexibly to accommodate new data forms and assay platforms.

Phase II: Assay Development and Validation

After the Phase I validity assessment, pathways would be selected for assay development. The focus would be on critical toxicity pathways that lead reliably to adverse effects for the organism and that are not secondary consequences of other biologic perturbations. The first section of this chapter outlined some of the technical issues that would require research to support assay development.

The case-study example of altered estrogen signaling above indicates how assays may follow from toxicity-pathway identification. Understanding the direct gene-regulation consequences of modulated ER-mediated transcriptional activation would lead to specific assays for quantitative assessment of transcription (RNA), translation (protein), metabolite markers, and altered function. Rapid assays to evaluate function on the scale of receptor activation of estrogen-mediated transcription of reporter genes or even estrogen-mediated cell responses, such as cell proliferation of estrogen-sensitive cells in vitro, could be developed to assess altered estrogen signaling.

Also important for assessing the potential for perturbations in estrogen signaling would be reliable assays for detecting estrogen receptor interactions rapidly. Specific assays that might be developed include ligand-receptor binding assays and more sophisticated computational structural models of ligand interactions with receptor and receptor-complex conformational changes. Further sets of assays would be needed to address the wide variety of toxicity pathways by which estrogenic compounds can operate. In this phase, biomarkers of effect, susceptibility, and exposure would be developed for use in human biomonitoring and surveillance.

Demonstrating that a test is reliable and relevant for a particular purpose is a prerequisite for its routine use for regulatory acceptance. But establishing the validity of any new toxicity assay can be a formidable process—expensive, time-consuming, and logistically and technically challenging. Development of efficient approaches for validating the new mechanistically based assays would add to the challenge. How can the assays come into use within a reasonable time and be sufficiently validated to be used with confidence? That question is discussed by considering first the relevant existing guidance on validation and then the challenges faced in validating the new tests. Finally, some general suggestions are made regarding validation of the new tests. In making its suggestions, the committee acknowledges the considerable work going on in institutions in the United States and Europe to improve validation methods.

Existing Validation Guidance

Guidelines on the validation of new and revised methods for regulatory acceptance have been developed by both regulatory agencies and consortia (ICCVAM/NICEAM 2003; OECD 2005). Such guidelines focus on multifactorial aspects of a test, which cover the following elements:

• Definition of test rationale, test components, and assay conduct and the provision of details on the test protocol.

• Consideration of the relationship of the test-method end points to the biologic effect of interest.

• Characterization of reproducibility in and among laboratories, transferability among laboratories, sources of variability, test limits, and other factors related to the reliability of test measurements (sometimes referred to as internal validity).

• Demonstrated biologic performance of the test with reference chemicals, comparison of the performance with that of the tests it is to replace, and description of test limitations (sometimes referred to as external validity).

• Availability, peer review, and good-laboratory-practices status of the data supporting the validation of the test method.

• Independent peer review of the methods and results of the test and publication in the peer-reviewed literature.

Criteria for regulatory acceptance of new test methods have also been published (ICCVAM/NICEAM 2003). They cover some of the subjects noted above and include criteria related to robustness (insensitivity to minor changes in protocol), time and cost effectiveness, capability of being harmonized and accepted by agencies and international groups, and capability of generating useful information for risk assessment.

Validation of a new test method typically is a prerequisite for regulatory acceptance but is no guarantee of acceptance. It establishes the performance characteristics of a test method for a particular purpose. Different regulatory agencies may decide that they have no need for a test intended for a given purpose, or they may set their criteria of acceptable performance higher or lower than other agencies. To minimize problems associated with acceptance, the Organisation for Economic Co-operation and Development (OECD 2005) recommends that validation and peer-review processes take place before a test is considered for acceptance as an OECD test guideline. OECD recognizes, however, that factors beyond the technical performance of an assay may be viewed differently by different regulatory authorities.

Challenges in Validating Mechanistically Based Assays

Validation of the mechanistically based tests envisioned by the committee may be especially challenging for several reasons. First, the tests in the new paradigm that are based on nonapical findings depart from current practice used by regulatory agencies in setting health advisories and guidelines based on apical outcomes. Relevant policy and legal issues are discussed at length in Chapter 6 and will not be repeated here except to note that scientific acceptance of a test and its relationship to disease is a critical component of establishment of the validity of the test for regulatory purposes.

Second, the new -omics and related technologies will need to be standardized and refined before specific applications can be validated for regulatory purposes (Corvi et al. 2006). Such preliminary work could be seen as an elaborate extension of the routine step of test-method optimization or prevalidation leading to validation of conventional in vivo or in vitro assays. The committee also notes above that some degree of standardization will be necessary early to promote understanding and use of assay findings by researchers for knowledge development.

Third, because -omics and related technologies are evolving rapidly, the decision to halt optimization of a particular application and begin a formal validation study will be somewhat subjective. Validation and regulatory acceptance of a specific test do not preclude incorporating later technologic advances that would enhance its performance. If it is warranted, the effects of such modifications on performance can be evaluated through an expedited validation that avoids the burdens of a second full-blown validation.

Fourth, the committee envisions that a suite of new tests typically will be needed to replace an individual in vivo test, given that apical findings can be triggered by multiple mechanisms. Consequently, although it is current practice to validate a single test against the corresponding conventional test and then to look for one-to-one correspondence, the new paradigm would routinely entail validation of test batteries and would use multivariate comparisons.

Fifth, existing validation guidelines focus on concordance between the results of the new and the existing assays. In practice, that often means comparing results from cell-based in vitro assays with in vivo data from animals. One of the challenges of validating the medium- and high-throughput assays in the new vision— with its emphasis on human-derived cells, cell lines, and cellular components—will be to identify standards of comparison for assessing their relevance and predictiveness while aiming for a transformative paradigm shift that emphasizes human biology, mechanisms of toxicity, and initial, critical perturbations of toxicity pathways.

Sixth, it is anticipated that virtually all xenobiotics will perturb signaling pathways to some degree, so a key challenge will be to determine when a perturbation leads to downstream toxicity and when it does not. Thus, specificity may be a bigger challenge than sensitivity.

Assay Validation under New Toxicity-Testing Paradigm

Validation should not be viewed as an inflexible process that proceeds sequentially through a fixed series of steps and is then judged according to unvarying criteria. For example, because validation assesses fitness for purpose, such exercises should be judged with the specific intended purpose in mind. A test's intended purpose may vary from use as a preliminary screening tool to use as the definitive test. Similarly, a new test may be intended to model one or a few toxicity mechanisms for a given apical end point but not the full array of mechanisms. Given that the new paradigm would emerge gradually, it would be important to consider validating incremental gains, while recognizing their current strengths and weaknesses.

Consequently, applying a one-size-fits-all approach to validation is not conducive to the rapid incorporation of emerging science or technology into regulatory decision-making. A more flexible approach to assay validation would facilitate the evolution of testing toward a more mechanistic understanding of toxicity end points; the form the validation should take is a point of discussion and deliberation (Balls et al. 2006; Corvi et al. 2006). For nonregulatory use of assays, preliminary data-gathering, and exploration of mechanisms, at a minimum some general guidance on assay performance appears warranted for intended assays. For assays to be used routinely, somewhat rigorous performance standards and relevance would have to be established.

Returning to the case study on estrogen signaling, the validation sequence involves the development of specific assays that track the key molecular triggers linked to human estrogenic effects. This validation component is largely focused first on validating that the assay components recapitulate the key molecular interactions above and then on the traditional approach of looking at assay performance in terms of reproducibility and relevance.

Assessing intralaboratory and interlaboratory reproducibility is more straightforward than assessing relevance, which is sometimes labeled accuracy. To assess relevance, assays would be formally linked to organism-level adverse health effects. For example, they would provide the basis of evaluating the level of molecular change that potentially corresponds to an adverse effect. In addition, reference compounds would be used to determine the assays' positive and negative predictive value. Ideally, substances known to cause and substances known not to cause the effect in humans would be used as the reference agents for positive and negative predictivity. In the absence of adequate numbers of xenobiotics known to be positive and negative in humans, animal data may have to be used in validation. For the assays based on human cell lines, that could be problematic, and some creativity and flexibility in the validation process would be desirable. For example, rodent-based cell assays comparable with the human assay could be used to establish relevance and support the use of the human cell-based assay.

Phase III: Assay Relevance and Validity Trial

Once assays are developed and formally validated, they would become available for use. The committee suggests three distinct strategies that could aid in the assessment of test validity and relevance and could further the development of improved assays.

First, research entities, such as the National Toxicology Program (NTP), should further develop and run the experimental high-throughput assays, some before they are fully validated, on chemicals that have already been extensively tested with standard or other toxicity tests. The NTP has, for example, initiated mechanistic high-throughput assays on at least 500 chemicals that have already been tested using NTP cancer and reproductive and developmental toxicity studies; and, in collaboration with the NIH Molecular Library Initiative, further developed and applied cell-based screening assays that can be automated (NTP 2006). The Environmental Protection Agency (EPA) National Center for Computational Toxicology (NCCT) also has an initiative to screen numerous pesticides and some industrial chemicals in high-throughput tests. Those processes would be essential for validating the new assays and for learning more about which health effects can be predicted from specific perturbations of toxicity pathways.

Second, new validated assays should be conducted in parallel with existing toxicity tests for chemicals, such as pesticides and pharmaceuticals, that will be undergoing or have recently undergone toxicity testing under regulatory programs. This research testing, which would be conducted by research entities, would help to foster the evolution of the assays into cell-based test batteries to eventually replace current tests. The testing would also help to gauge the positive and negative predictive values of the various assays and thereby help to avoid (or at least begin to quantify) the associated risks with missing important toxicities with the new assays or incorporating a new assay that detects meaningless physiologic alterations that are not useful for predicting human risk.

Third, as the new assays are developed further and validated, they should be deployed as screens for evaluation of chemicals that would not currently undergo toxicity testing, such as existing high-production-volume chemicals that have not been tested or have been evaluated only with the screening information dataset, or new chemicals that are not currently subject to test requirements. Used as screens for chemicals that would otherwise not be tested or be subject only to little testing, the assays could begin to help to set priorities for testing and could also help to guide the focus of any testing that may be required. Eventually they could provide the basis of an improved framework for addressing chemicals for which testing is limited or not done at all. This is illustrated in Figure 5-2.

Resources will be required to implement the three approaches: testing of chemicals with large and robust datasets of apical tests, parallel research testing of chemicals subject to existing regulatory testing requirements, and applying high-through-

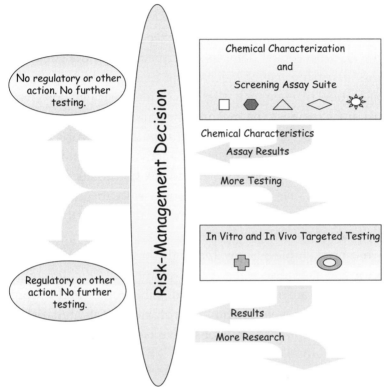

FIGURE 5-2 Screening of chemicals that would otherwise not be tested or be subject to only limited testing. The results of the screening tests would be used to decide the nature of further testing needed, if any.

put screens to chemicals that are currently not tested. In making those suggestions, the committee is not recommending expanding test requirements for pesticides or pharmaceuticals. Rather, it notes that the tests developed will be a national resource of wide benefit and worthy of funding by federal research programs. Voluntary testing by industry using validated new assays should also be encouraged. The three approaches are anticipated to pay off substantially in the longer term as scientists, regulators, and stakeholders develop enough familiarity and comfort with the new assays that they begin to replace current apical end-point tests and as mechanistic indicators are increasingly used in environmental decision-making.

In addition to the high-throughput testing by NTP and EPA of chemicals with robust datasets described above, the committee notes the increasing use of mechanistic assays, primarily for further evaluation of chemicals that have demonstrated toxicity in standard apical assays. The mechanistic studies are done to evaluate further a tailored subset of toxicity pathways, such as those involving the peroxisome proliferators-activated receptor, the aryl hydrocarbon receptor, and thyroid and sex hormones. Some companies are also using high-throughput assays to guide internal decision-making in new chemical development, but their results typically are not publicly available.

A recent example of how the high-throughput assays could play out in the near term is the risk assessment of perchlorate. The data on perchlorate include standard subchronic- and chronic-toxicity tests and developmental-neurotoxicity tests, but risk assessments and regulatory decisions have been based on perturbation of iodide-uptake inhibition—the known toxicity pathway through which perchlorate has its effects (EPA 2006; NRC 2006). If a new chemical were found to inhibit iodide uptake, standard toxicity tests would not be necessary to demonstrate the predictable effects on thyroid hormone and neurodevelopment. Regulatory decisions could be based on the dose-response relationship for iodide-uptake inhibition. The new data on perchlorate-susceptible subpopulations (for example, those with low iodide) emerging from biomonitoring would also be considered (see Blount et al. 2006). Such a chemical would need to undergo a full battery of toxicity-pathway testing to ascertain that no other important pathways that might have effects at lower doses were disrupted.

In the long run, using upstream indicators of toxicity from high-throughput assays based on toxicity pathways can be more sensitive and hence more protective of public health then using apical-end-point observations from assays in small numbers of live rodents. However, while the new assays are under development, there will be a long period of uncertainty during which the false-positive and false-negative rates of the testing battery will remain unclear, and the ability of the battery to adequately predict effects in susceptible subpopulations or during susceptible life stages will also be unclear. During the phase-in period and afterward, there will be a need to pay close attention to whether important toxicities are being missed or are being exaggerated by the toxicity-pathway screening battery. The concern about missing important toxic end points is one of the main reasons for the committee's recommendation for a long phase-in period during which the new assays are run in parallel with existing assays and tested on chemicals on which there are already large robust datasets of apical findings. Parallel testing will allow identification of toxicities that might be missed if the new assays were used alone and will compel the development of assays to address these gaps.

Many additional issues would need to be considered during the interim phase of assay development. For example, technical issues, such as cell-culture conditions, and selective pressures that result in molecular evolution of cell lines over time and across laboratories could result in issues that could be addressed only with experience and careful review of assay results. Parallel use of new assays and current tests would probably continue for some time before the adoption of the new assays as first-tier screens or as definitive tests of toxicity.

Phase IV: Assembly and Validation of Test Batteries

Once toxicity pathways are elucidated and translated into high-throughput assays for a broad field of toxicity testing, such as neurotoxicology, a progressively more comprehensive suite of validated medium- to high-throughput tests would become available to cover the field. Single assays would not be comprehensive or predictive in isolation but would be assembled into suites with targeted tests that would cover the field. The suite or "panel" of assays and the scoring of the assays would need to be assessed. This may involve a computational assessment of multivariate end points. Turning again to the estrogen-signaling case study, known estrogen modulators should register as positive in one or more assays. Confidence in the suite of assays can come from the knowledge that all known mechanisms of estrogenic-signaling alteration are modeled.

The development and assessment of batteries and the overall testing strategy would be facilitated by a formal uncertainty evaluation. For the different risk contexts and decisions to be made (Chapter 3), the preferred test batteries may differ in sensitivity, in this context the probability that the battery identifies as harmful a dose that is harmful, and specificity, the probability that a test battery identifies as not harmful a dose that is not harmful. In screening, the effect of a false-negative finding of no harm at a given dose can be far more costly than a false-positive finding of harm (see, for example, Lave and Omenn 1986). The ability to characterize the specificity and sensitivity of the test battery would aid the consideration of the cost effectiveness and value of the information to be obtained from the test battery (Lave and Omenn 1986; Lave et al. 1988) and ultimately help to identify preferred test strategies.

Although considerable effort would be directed at the construction of high-throughput batteries, targeted tests would probably also be needed in routine testing strategies to address particular risk contexts (for example, registration of a pesticide for food uses). Still, the end-point-focused targeted assays should by no means remain static. Instead, they should evolve to incorporate new refinements. For example, the rapid developments in imaging technologies have offered scientists important new tools to enhance the collection of information from animal bioassays. Promising new assays that use nonmammalian models, such as

Caenorhabditis elegans, are in development. Combined mammalian assays that incorporate a broader array of sensitive end points in a more efficient manner have been developed. The committee assumes that development of those approaches will continue, and it encourages development and validation of them in targeted testing. As newer targeted-testing approaches become available, older apical approaches should be retired.

Intermediate Products of Assay-Development Research

One important benefit of the research described is that it could add public-health protection and refinement to current regulatory testing. For example, in some risk contexts, particularly widespread human exposure to existing chemicals, the dose-response data from toxicity-pathway tests could help to refine quantitative relationships between adverse effects identified in the apical tests and perturbations in toxicity pathways and improve the evaluation of perturbations at the low end of the dose-response curve. The results of the toxicity-pathway tests could provide data to aid in interpreting the results of apical tests on a given substance and may guide the selection of further follow-up tests or epidemiologic surveillance. The mechanistic assays would also help to permit the extrapolation of toxicity findings on a chemical under study to other chemicals that target the same mechanism. Additional benefits and research products anticipated for use in the near term include the following:

• A battery of inexpensive medium- and high-throughput screening assays that could be incorporated into tiered-testing schemes to identify the most appropriate tests or to provide preliminary results for screening risk assessments. With experience, the assays would support the phase-out of apical end-point tests.

- Early cell-based replacements for some in vivo tests, such as those for acute toxicity.
- Work to develop consensus approaches for DNA-reactivity and mutagenicity assays and strategies for using mechanistic studies in cancer risk assessment.
- On-line libraries of results of medium- and high-throughput screens for use in toxicity prediction and improving SAR models. For classes of chemicals well studied in apical end-point tests, the comparison of results from high-throughput studies with those from whole-animal studies could provide the basis of extrapolating toxicity to untested chemicals in the class.
- Elucidation of the mechanisms of toxicity of chemicals well studied in high-dose apical end-point tests. Research to achieve the vision must include the study of perturbations of toxicity pathways of well-studied chemicals, many of which have widespread human exposure. Such research would bring about better understanding of the mechanisms of toxicity of the chemicals and improve risk assessment. Chemicals with known adverse effects and mechanisms well elucidated with respect to toxicity pathways would be good candidates to serve as positive controls in the high-throughput assays. Such studies would help to distinguish between exposures that result in impaired function and disease and exposures that result in adaptation and normal biologic function (see Figure 2-2).
- Indicators of toxicity-pathway activation in the human population. This knowledge could be used to understand the extent to which a single chemical might contribute to disease processes and would be critical for realistic dose-response modeling and extrapolation.
- Refined analytic tools for assessing the pharmacokinetics of environmental agents in humans exposed at low concentrations. Such evaluations could be used directly in risk assessments based on apical end-point tests and could aid in design and interpretation of in vitro screens.

- Improvements in targeted human disease surveillance and exposure biomonitoring.

BUILDING A TRANSFORMATIVE RESEARCH PROGRAM

Instituting Focused Research

A long-term, large-scale concerted effort is needed to bring the new toxicity-testing paradigm to fruition. A critical element is the conduct of transformative research to provide the scientific basis of creating the new testing tools and to understand the implications of test results and how they may be applied in risk assessments used in environmental decision-making.

What type of institutional structure would be most appropriate for conducting and managing the research effort? It is beyond the committee's charge and expertise to make specific recommendations either to change or to create government institutions or to alter their funding decisions. The committee will simply sketch its thoughts on an appropriate institutional structure for implementing the vision. Other approaches may also be appropriate.

The committee notes that an institutional structure should be selected with the following considerations in mind:

- The realization of the vision will entail considerable research over many years and require substantial funding—hundreds of millions of dollars.
- Much of the research will be interdisciplinary and consequently, to be most effective, should not be dispersed among discipline-specific laboratories.
- The research will need high-level coordination to tackle the challenges presented in the vision efficiently.
- The research should be informed by the needs of the regulatory agencies that would adapt and use the emerging testing

procedures, but the research program should be insulated from the short-term orientation and varied mandates of the agencies.

Interdisciplinarity, Adaptability, and Timeline

The need for an institutional structure that encourages and coordinates the necessarily multidisciplinary research cannot be overstated, and a spirit of interdisciplinarity should infuse the research program. Accordingly, the effort would need to draw on a variety of technologies and a number of disciplines, including basic biology, bioinformatics, biostatistics, chemistry, computational biology, developmental biology, engineering, epidemiology, genetics, pathology, structural biology, and toxicology. Good communication and problem-solving across disciplines are a must, as well as leadership adept at fostering interdisciplinary efforts. The effort will have to be monitored continually, with the necessary cross-interactions engineered, managed, and maintained.

The testing paradigm would be progressively elaborated over many years or decades as experience and successes accumulate. It should continue to evolve with scientific advances. Its evolution is likely to entail midcourse changes in the direction of research as breakthroughs in technology and science open more promising leads. Neither this committee nor any other constituted committee will be able to foresee the full suite of possibilities or potential limitations of new approaches that might arise with increasing biologic knowledge. The research strategy outlined above provides a preview to the future and suggests general steps needed to arrive at a new toxicity-testing paradigm. Some of the suggested steps would need to be reconsidered as time passes and experience is developed with new cell-based assays and interpretive tools, but no global change in the vision, which the committee regards as robust, is expected.

The transition from existing tests to the new tests would require active management, involvement of the regulatory agencies, and coherent long-range planning that invests in the creation of new knowledge while refining current testing and, correspondingly, stimulating changes in risk-assessment procedures and guidelines. Over time, the research expertise and infrastructure involved in testing regimes could be transformed in important ways as the need for animal testing decreases and pathway-related testing increases.

The committee envisions that the new knowledge and technology generated from the proposed research program will be translated to noticeable changes in toxicity-testing practices within 10 years. Within 20 years, testing approaches will more closely reflect the proposed vision than current approaches. That projection assumes adequate and sustained funding. As in the Human Genome Project, progress is expected to be nonlinear, with the pace increasing as technologic and scientific breakthroughs are applied to the effort.

Cross-Institution and Sector Linkages

The research to describe cellular-response networks and toxicity pathways and to develop the complementary human bio-monitoring and surveillance strategy would be part of larger current efforts in medicine and biotechnology. Funding of that research is substantial in medical schools and other academic institutions, some U.S. federal and European agencies, and pharmaceutical, medical, and biotechnology industries. Links among different elements in the research community involved in relevant research will be needed to capitalize on the new knowledge, technologies, and analytic tools as they develop. Mechanisms for ensuring sustained communication and collaboration, such as data-sharing, will also be needed.

Some form of participation by industry and public-interest groups should be ensured. Firms have a long-term interest in the new paradigm, and most stand to gain from more efficient testing requirements. Public-health and environmental interest groups, as well as those promoting alternatives to animal testing, should also be engaged.

Funding

A large-scale, long-term research program is needed to elucidate the cellular-response networks and individual toxicity pathways within them. Given the scientific challenges and knowledge development required, moderately large funding will be required. The committee envisions a research and test-development program similar in scale to the NTP or the Institute for Systems Biology in Seattle, Washington.

The success of the project will depend on attracting the best thinkers to the task, and the endeavor would compete with related research programs in medicine, industry, and government for these researchers. Attracting the best researchers in turn would depend on an adequately funded and managed venture that appears well placed to succeed.

Institutional Framework

The committee concludes that an appropriate institutional structure for the proposed vision is a research institute that fosters multidisciplinary research intramurally and extramurally. A strong intramural research program is essential. The effort cannot succeed merely by creating a virtual institution to link and integrate organizations that are performing relevant research and by dispersing funding on relevant research projects. A mission-oriented, intramural program with core multidisciplinary programs to answer the critical research questions can foster the kind of cross-discipline activity essential for the success of the initiative. There would be far less chance of success within a reasonable period if the research were dispersed among different locations and organizations without a core integrating and organizing institute. A collocated, strong intramural research initiative will enable the communication and problem-solving across disciplines required for the research and assay development.

Similarly, a strong, well-coordinated, targeted extramural program will leverage the expertise that already exists within academe, pharmaceutical companies, the biotechnology sector, and elsewhere and foster research that complements the intramural program. Through its intramural and highly targeted extramural activities, the envisioned research institute would provide the nexus through which the new testing tools would be conceived, developed, validated, and incorporated into coherent testing schemes.

The committee sees the research institute funded and coordinated primarily by the federal government, given the scale of the necessary funding, the multiyear nature of the project, and links to government regulatory agencies. That does not mean that there will be no role for other stakeholders. Biotechnology companies, for example, could cofund specific projects. Academic researchers could conduct research with the program's extramural funds. Moreover, researchers in industry and academe will continue making important progress in fields related to the proposed vision independently of the proposed projects.

The key institutional question is where to house the government research institute that carries out the intramural program of core multidisciplinary research and manages the extramural program of research. Should it be an existing entity, such as the National Institute of Environmental Health Sciences (NIEHS), or a new entity devoted exclusively to the proposed vision? The committee notes that the recognized need for research and institutional structures that transcend disciplinary boundaries to address critical biomedical research questions has spawned systems-biology institutes and centers at biomedical firms and several leading universities in the country. However, the committee found few examples in the government sector. The Department of Energy (DOE) Genomics GTL Program seeks to engineer systems for energy production, site remediation, and carbon sequestration based on systems-biology research on microorganisms. In its review of this DOE program, NRC (2006) found collocated, integrated vertical research to be essential to its success.

If one were to place the proposed research program into an existing government entity, a possible choice would be the NTP, a multiagency entity administered and housed in NIEHS. The NTP has several features that suggest it as a possible institutional home for the research program envisioned here, including its mandate to develop innovative testing approaches, its multiagency character, the similarities between its Vision and Roadmap for the Future and what is envisioned here, and its expertise in validating new tests through the NTP Interagency Center for the Evaluation of Alterative Toxicological Methods and its sister entity, the Interagency Coordinating Committee on the Validation of Alternative Methods, and in -omics testing at its Center for Toxicogenomics. It is conceivable that the NTP could absorb the research mandate outlined here if its efforts dramatically scaled up to accommodate the focused program envisioned. If it were placed in the NTP, structures would have to be in place to ensure that the day-to-day technical focus on short-term problems of high-volume chemical testing would not impede progress in evolving testing strategies. As the new test batteries and strategies are developed and validated, they would be moved out of the research arm and be made available for routine application.

The committee considered housing the proposed research institute in a regulatory agency and notes that this could be problematic. The science and technology budgets of regulatory agencies have been under considerable stress and appear unlikely to sustain such an effort. Although EPA's NCCT has initiated important work in this field, the scale of the endeavor envisioned by the committee is substantially larger and could not be sufficiently supported if recent trends in congressional budgeting for EPA continue. For example, EPA's science and technology research budget has been suboptimal and decreasing in real dollars for a number of years (EPA 2006, 2007).

The research portfolio entailed by the committee's vision will also require active management to maintain relevance and the scientific focus needed for knowledge development. Although sufficient input from regulatory agencies is needed, insulation of the institute from the short-term orientation of regulatory-agency programs that depend on the results of toxicologic testing is important.

In the end, the committee noted that wherever the institute is housed, it should be structured along the lines of the NTP, with intramural and focused extramural components and interagency input but with its own focused mission and funding stream.

Scientific Surprises and the Need for Midcourse Corrections

Research often brings surprises, and today's predictions concerning the promise of particular lines of research are probably either pessimistic or optimistic in some details. For example, the committee's vision of toxicity testing stands on the presumption that a relatively small number of pathways can provide sufficiently broad coverage to allow a moderately sized set of high- and medium-throughput assays to be developed for the scientific community to use with confidence and that any important gaps in coverage can be addressed with a relatively small set of targeted assays. That presumption may be found to be incorrect. Furthermore, the establishment of links between perturbations and apical end points may prove especially challenging for some end points. Thus, as the research proceeds and learning takes place, adjustments in the vision and the research focus can be anticipated.

In addition to program oversight noted above, the research program should be assessed every 3-5 years by well-recognized scientific experts independently of vested interests in the public and private sectors. The assessment would weigh practical progress, the promise of methods on the research horizon, and the place of the research in the context of other research, and it would recommend midcourse corrections.

CONCLUDING REMARKS

In the traditional approach to toxicity testing, the whole animal provides for the integration and evaluation of many toxicity pathways. Yet each animal study is time-consuming and expensive and results in the use of many animals. In addition, many animal studies need to be done to evaluate different end points, life stages, and exposure durations. The new approach may require individual assays for hundreds of relevant toxicity pathways. Despite that apparent complexity, emerging methods allow testing of many pathways extremely rapidly and efficiently (for example, in microarrays or wells). If positive signals from the assays can be used with confidence to guide risk management, the new approach will ultimately prove more efficient than the traditional one.

It is clear, however, that much development and refinement will be needed before a new and efficient system could be in place. For some kinds of toxicity, such as developmental toxicity and neurotoxicity, the identification of replacement toxicity-pathway assays might be particularly challenging, and some degree of targeted testing might continue to be necessary. In addition, the validation process may uncover unexpected and challenging technical problems that will require targeted testing. Finally, the parallel interim process may discover that some categories of chemicals or of toxicity cannot yet be evaluated with toxicity-pathway testing. Nonetheless, the committee envisions the steady evolution of toxicity testing from apical end-point testing to a system based largely on toxicity-pathway batteries in a manner mindful of information needs and of the capacity of the test system to provide information.

In the long term, the committee expects toxicity pathways to become sufficiently well understood and calibrated for batteries of high-throughput assays to provide a substantial fraction of the toxicity-testing data needed for environmental decision-making. Exposure monitoring, human surveillance for early perturbations of toxicity-response pathways, and epidemiologic studies should provide an additional layer of assurance that early indications of adverse effects would be detected if they occurred. The research conducted to realize the committee's vision would support a series of substantial improvements in toxicity testing in the relatively near term.

REFERENCES

Balls, M., P. Amcoff, S. Bremer, S. Casati, S. Coecke, R. Clothier, R. Combes, R. Corvi, R. Curren, C. Eskes, J. Fentem, L. Gribaldo, M. Halder, T. Hartung, S. Hoffmann, L. Schectman, L. Scott, H. Spielmann, W. Stokes, R. Tice, D. Wagner, and V. Zuang. 2006. The principles of weight of evidence validation of test methods and testing strategies. The report and recommendations of ECVAM workshop 58. Altern. Lab. Anim. 34(6):603-620.

Blount, B.C., J.L. Pirkle, J.D. Osterloh, L. Valentin-Blasini, and K.L. Caldwell. 2006. Urinary perchlorate and thyroid hormone levels in adolescent and adult men and women living in the United States. Environ. Health Perspect. 114(12):1865–1871.

Brazma, A., P. Hingamp, J. Quackenbush, G. Sherlock, P. Spellman, C. Stoeckert, J. Aach, W. Ansorge, C.A. Ball, H.C. Causton, T. Gaasterland, P. Glenisson, F.C. Holstege, I.F. Kim, V. Markowitz, C. Matese, H. Parkinson, A.

Robinson, U. Sarkans, S. Schulze-Kremer, J. Stewart, R. Taylor, J. Vilo, and M. Vingron. 2001. Minimum information about a microarray experiment (MIAME)-toward standards for microarray data. Nat. Genet. 29(4):365-371.

Corvi, R., H.J. Ahr, S. Albertini, D.H. Blakey, L. Clerici, S. Coecke, G.R. Douglas, L. Gribaldo, J.P. Groten, B. Haase, K. Hamernik, T. Hartung, T. Inoue, I. Indans, D. Maurici, G. Orphanides, D. Rembges, S.A. Sansone, J.R. Snape, E. Toda, W. Tong, J.H. van Delft, B. Weis, and L.M. Schechtman. 2006. Meeting report: Validation of toxicogenomics-based test systems: ECVAM-ICCVAM/NICEATM considerations for regulatory use. Environ Health Perspect. 114(3):420-429.

EPA (U.S. Environmental Protection Agency). 2006. Science and Research Budgets for the U.S. Environmental Protection Agency for Fiscal Year 2007; An Advisory Report by the Science Advisory Board. EPA-SAB-ADV-06-003. U.S. Environmental Protection Agency, Washington DC. March 30, 2006 [online]. Available: http://yosemite.epa.gov/sab/sabproduct.nsf/36a1ca3f683ae57a85256ce9006a32d0/0EDAAECA1096A5B085257145007 2E33E/$File/sab-adv-06-003.pdf [accessed April 4, 2007].

EPA (U.S. Environmental Protection Agency). 2007. Comments on EPA's Strategic Research Directions and Research Budget for FY 2008, An Advisory Report of the U.S. Environmental Protection Agency Science Advisory Board. EPA-SAB-ADV-07-004. U.S. Environmental Protection Agency, Washington DC. March 13, 2007 [online]. Available: http://yosemite.epa.gov/sab/sabproduct.nsf/997517EFA5FC48798525729F00 73B4D4/$File/sab-07-004.pdf [accessed April 7, 2007].

ICCVAM (Interagency Coordinating Committee on the Validation of Alternative Methods) and NICEATM (National Toxicology Program Interagency Center for the Evaluation of Alternative Toxicolgical Methods). 2003. ICCVAM Guidelines for the Nomination and Submission of New, Revised, and Alternative Test Methods. NIH Publication No. 03-4508. National Institute of Environmental Health Sciences, National Institutes of Health.

Inglese, J., D.S. Auld, A. Jadhav, R.L. Johnson, A. Simeonov, A. Yasgar, W. Zheng, and C.P. Austin. 2006. Quantitative high-throughput screening: A titration-based approach that efficiently identifies biological activities in large chemical libraries. Proc. Natl. Acad. Sci. U.S.A. 103(31):11473-11478.

Lave, L.B., and G.S. Omenn. 1986. Cost-effectiveness of short-term tests for carcinogenicity. Nature 324(6092):29-34.

Lave, L.B., F.K. Ennever, H.S. Rosenkranz, and G.S. Omenn. 1988. Information value of the rodent bioassay. Nature 336(6200):631-633.

NRC (National Research Council). 2000. Scientific Frontiers in Developmental Toxicology and Risk Assessment. Washington, DC: National Academy Press.

NRC (National Research Council). 2006. Review of the Department of Energy's Genomics: GTL Program. Washington, DC: The National Academies Press.
NTP (National Toxicology Program). 2006. Current Directions and Evolving Strategies. National Toxicology Program, National Institute of Environmental Health Sciences, National Institutes of Health, Research Triangle Park, NC[online]. Available: http://ntp.niehs.nih.gov/files/NTP_CurrDir2006.pdf [accessed April 4, 2007].
OECD (Organisation for Economic Co-operation and Development). 2005. Guidance Document on the Validation and International Acceptance of New or Updated Test Methods for Hazard Assessment. OECD Series on Testing and Assessment No. 34. ENV/JM/Mono(2005)14. Organisation for Economic Co-operation and Development, Paris [online]. Available: http://appli1.oecd.org/olis/2005doc.nsf/linkto/env-jm-mono(2005)14 [accessed April 4, 2007].

6

Prerequisites for Implementing the Vision in Regulatory Contexts

The committee's vision sets the stage for transformative changes in toxicity testing in the regulatory agencies and the larger scientific community. Although advances in the state of the science are indispensable to realization of the vision, corresponding institutional changes are also important. The changes will promote acceptance of the principles and methods envisioned. Acceptance will depend on several factors, some having scientific origins. For example, the new testing requirements will be expected to reflect the state of the science and to be founded on peer-reviewed research, established protocols, validated models, case examples, and other scientific features. Other factors stem from administrative procedures associated with rule-making, such as documenting scientific sources; providing opportunities for scientific experts, stakeholders, and the interested public to participate; and consulting with sister agencies and international organizations.

This chapter explores the conditions required for using the new testing strategy for regulatory purposes. It focuses on the federal agencies and identifies institutional outlooks and orientation—both tangible, such as budget and staffing, and intangible, such as leadership and commitment—that can determine the pace and degree to which the vision is incorporated into agency culture and practice. The chapter also addresses the fundamental issues related to the use and the validity of the new concepts, technologies, and resulting data for the specific purpose of developing federal regulations.

The committee's vision anticipates continual change over the next 2-3 decades. Beyond the scientific and procedural considerations summarized in this chapter, the state of the economy, changing environmental conditions and social perspectives, and other dynamics that shape the political climate will influence legislative changes and federal budgets that, in turn, will determine the future of toxicity testing in the regulatory context.

INSTITUTIONAL CHANGE TO MEET THE VISION

Attitudes and Expectations

Full realization of the vision depends on the promotion of new testing principles and methods in the scientific community at large. As in the past, some changes will originate outside the regulatory agencies and work their way into agency practice, and others will originate in the agencies and work their way into the larger scientific community. In both cases, far-reaching shifts in orientation and perception will be critical. For risk assessors and researchers, the shifts will be from familiar types of studies and established procedures involving overt effects in laboratory animals and cross-species extrapolation to new approaches that focus on how chemicals, both endogenous and exogenous, interact in human disease processes (Lieber 2006). Many analysts in and outside the agencies will have to apply their expertise in new ways.

The need for a change in attitude and orientation extends far beyond risk assessors and the toxicity-testing community. Most difficult, perhaps, will be the new level of scientific understanding needed to enable many participants, especially nonscientists, to become sufficiently informed to engage in discussion of the new methods. Law-makers who determine policy and appropriate funds, federal executives who determine research priorities, politically accountable managers and decision-makers who use data-based risk assessment for making regulatory decisions, courts that review those decisions, and the public, which has an interest in the need for and nature of regulations, will need to become acquainted with new terminology and concepts.

Nonscientists will grasp some aspects of the new science— such as having regulations based on data derived from human cells, cell lines, and tissues rather than on laboratory animals— more easily than other aspects, such as the molecular basis of chemical changes that lead to adverse health effects. Ideally, individual or institutional "champions" will emerge to foster and guide the implementation process.

Developing and Cultivating Expertise

Effective implementation depends on competent scientists and informed agency management. Those factors are crucial: agency progress depends on the expertise and experience of the technical staff and a supportive management structure. Incorporating new tests and testing strategies into risk-assessment practices and agency testing guidelines will go no further or faster than staffing permits.

For several decades, academic institutions have prepared scientists for toxicity testing and risk analysis through training in chemistry, biology, toxicology, pharmacology, and the related medical and engineering disciplines. Agency scientists receive their basic undergraduate and postgraduate education and training from external institutions and bring their training to bear on their work for the agencies. For many, pre-agency experience includes postdoctoral fellowships, internships, or first jobs at universities, industry laboratories, consulting laboratories, and other outside organizations. The kind of expertise currently available in the agencies therefore reflects in large measure expertise in the larger scientific community. That tradition has contributed to a large and stable cadre of well-trained scientists in the federal agencies that have science-based responsibilities. Thus, implementing the vision will require an infusion of new scientists who have education and experience in the new technologies and special training for current scientific staff and managers.

Scientists in academe, industry, and consulting laboratories and organizations have had a productive exchange with those in regulatory agencies through professional conferences and workshops, joint research projects, and peer-review activities. Fostering and accelerating those activities will be critical for implementing the vision and will require congressional and management support of targeted investment in developing and sustaining agency expertise. Scientists gravitate to attractive, well-funded, and well-staffed programs. To hire and retain high-caliber scientists in the numbers and disciplines needed, agencies will need congressional and management support of the vision reflected in budget allocations and hiring authorizations.

Policies to Foster Development and Use of New Tests

Institutional change does not come easily. The history of toxicity testing indicates that the pace and extent of change will depend in part on policies and incentives. Some policies and incentives to encourage the use and development of the new tests by agencies are discussed here.

First, continued progress in the use of the new technologies constitutes the greatest incentive to reconfiguring agency testing programs in line with the vision. Policies to support and reward effective use of new testing concepts and methods should be implemented. Apart from historical high-visibility examples, such as the Human Genome Project, current broad-scale examples include the development and use of mechanistic data and the expanding list of –omics applications.

Second, policies to encourage the use of data generated with the new testing paradigm in chemical assessments by the agencies will be important. That will involve the evolution of agencies' risk-assessment methods and guidelines as the new tests are developed and used. For decades, the federal agencies have promulgated formal risk-assessment guidelines, based in part on consultation with outside scientists and the public, that codify generally accepted concepts and methods to be followed in assessing the hazards, dose-response relationships, exposures, and risks related to environmental agents (for example, EPA 1991, 1996, 1998a, 2005). Policies to include the new technologies in agency assessments can foster and accelerate their acceptance and institutionalization.

Third, congressional funding of agencies to implement the vision is essential to support relevant research and staffing, encourage work with external scientists outside the agencies, recognize accomplishments by scientists and their management, and support other policies to promote change.

Fourth, dependence of market access on the conduct of specific toxicity tests can be a policy incentive. For example, the European Union's Registration, Evaluation and Authorisation of Chemicals (REACH) program requires generation of a basic set of toxicity data on new industrial chemicals before the chemicals can enter the market; the program also sets deadlines for receipt of basic toxicity data on existing industrial chemicals. Another example is the registration of pesticides in the United States.

Fifth, scientific progress in toxicity testing depends on work in academic and private-sector laboratories and in the federal sector. Congressional and agency policies and activities must ensure that sufficiently informative data generated from effective new methods are used in the regulatory process and that the large expenditures of money are not in vain.

Sixth, policies designed to overcome tendencies to resist novel approaches and maintain the status quo will be important. Implementing the vision requires periodic re-examination of testing programs and strategies in each agency and possibly a return to Congress to address outdated and ineffective programs that might impede implementation of novel tests and improved testing strategies.

REGULATORY USE OF NEW METHODS

The committee's vision sets the stage for transformative change in developing data to meet regulatory objectives codified in laws passed by Congress. Although the term *toxicity testing* rarely, if ever, appears in the major statutes administered by the U.S. Environmental Protection Agency (EPA), the availability of reliable data on "adverse effects" and health or environmental "risk" is an underlying assumption in them. The Clean Water Act, the Clean Air Act, the Toxic Substances Control Act (TSCA), and pesticide and Superfund legislation are based on the availability of data for risk assessment and regulatory decision-making for chemicals in their jurisdictions.

The data can have several sources. Some statutes—such as the Federal Insecticide, Fungicide, and Rodenticide Act (FIFRA), the Food Quality Protection Act, and TSCA—authorize EPA to require the producers of some chemicals to develop and submit specific categories of data to the agency. Other statutes—such as the Clean Air Act, the Clean Water Act, and the Safe Drinking Water Act—require toxicity data to be considered but depend mainly on information available in the scientific literature or government laboratory reports.[1] Regardless of the statute or the data source, toxicity data are indispensable for well-reasoned conclusions on the nature and dimensions of risk and for well-grounded decisions on the necessity of regulation to protect the public health or the environment and on the nature and scope of any such regulations.

As discussed in previous chapters, the committee's vision will result in the generation of data on perturbations in toxicity pathways with the use of high- and medium-throughput assays. A few of the test methods considered in this report have a long history and a place in the current regulatory testing programs and current risk-assessment guidelines and practices. Others are in early stages of development and have yet to be considered for regulatory use. Still others that will be used eventually are not yet on the drawing board or even imagined. Debate on the scientific validity of nonapical test methods and the application of the resulting data should be expected, and controversy could stall or bar the use of new test methods by regulatory agencies.

The discussion here addresses the prospect of controversy and focuses on the validity and defensibility of the new approaches. The primary measure of validity for regulatory purposes is scientific validity. Evidence of reliability and credibility that satisfies established scientific criteria is the principal basis for adopting and adapting new testing concepts and methods for regulatory use.[2] However, there are also policy and procedural

---

[1]In some cases, these statutes authorize EPA to apply TSCA and FIFRA testing requirements to chemicals in their jurisdiction.

[2]_Validity_ in this sense does not require de novo testing or further confirmation of previously validated scientific tests (see Chapter 5). Rather, it involves producing documentary evidence that the tests have been validated consistently with

aspects to validation, so the discussion also addresses administrative policies and procedures and other nonscientific considerations related to promulgating and defending government testing practices and requirements.[3]

Scientific Prerequisites of Validity

The federal agencies have a 75-year history of developing and promulgating toxicity-testing requirements for external entities, such as pesticide and drug manufacturers, and internal guidance for government laboratories (see Chapter 1). Documenting the validity, reliability, and relevance of test methods to the satisfaction of the scientific community has been and will continue to be an essential first step in identifying appropriate methods for use in the regulatory context. That documentation can also provide information and a tutorial for decision-makers, the public, and the courts.

Individual agency testing requirements do not arise de novo. For example, EPA's Office of Pesticide Programs promulgates test guidelines and requirements only after a comprehensive development and review process involving public comment, harmonization with other international organizations, and peer review by experts in the field.[4] Documentary evidence of validity has many sources and takes several forms. It includes evidence that customary criteria of scientific acceptance, such as peer review and publication in scholarly journals, have been satisfied. Use by other laboratories, other government agencies, or international organizations, such as the Organisation for Economic Co-operation and

---

standard scientific criteria. The objective is to avoid bringing unproven tests and the resulting data into the regulatory system.

[3]New data and data categories developed in line with the proposed changes in testing can be expected to affect many aspects of risk assessment and risk management. This section comments mainly on testing requirements.

[4]See, for example, 63 Fed. Reg. 41845-41848 (1998) and EPA 2006.

Development, is an indication of scientific acceptability. As new methods emerge, case studies and peer-reviewed testing guidelines, standardized operating procedures, and practice can be used to document validity.

Establishing and documenting the validity of the new nonapical test methods and the validity of markers of adverse responses corresponding to perturbations of toxicity pathways will be important milestones in implementing the committee's vision for regulatory use. Some considerations for accomplishing this are discussed below.

Adopting and Adapting New Test Systems and Methods

The vision prompts questions regarding the extent to which scientific progress using primarily human cells, cell lines, and cellular components in vitro can replace and, ideally, surpass in vivo mammalian systems as predictors of toxic effects in humans. Testing with cellular systems derived from human tissue and from nonmammalian systems is backed by an impressive scientific literature and has a long history that includes major contributions to cancer research and the Human Genome Project.

Regulatory agencies also use in vitro systems for toxicity testing and risk assessment. In vitro mode-of-action data were central elements when EPA proposed revisions to the cancer guidelines more than 10 years ago and in the final guidelines (EPA 2005). Mode-of-action data are featured in a wide array of risk assessments in EPA, other government institutions, and the private sector (for example, Meek et al. 2003; CalEPA 2004; NTP 2005; IARC 2006). EPA's exploration of mode-of-action approaches illustrates the use of information on biologic perturbations involved in key toxicity pathways.

With few exceptions, such studies are used in the regulatory context mainly to supplement or complement data from in vivo studies. As a result, despite the established value of in vitro systems for many purposes, increased reliance on them for regulatory testing may require further evidence of validity. As discussed in this report, a particularly important aspect of establishing validity concerns metabolism. Many of the issues are highlighted in the following statement:

> Several major problems are encountered in studying metabolism-related toxicity in vitro: (a) modeling human metabolism...; (b) maintaining tissue-specific function in vitro; (c) selecting an appropriate xenobiotic metabolizing system; (d) keeping enzyme activity stable over time; and (e) the adverse effects to toxicity-indicator cells of subcellular metabolizing fractions. . . . Two further problems [are] the testing of mixtures of chemicals that might require different enzyme systems . . . and . . . the inactivation of exogenous biotransformation systems, due to exposure to certain solvents and test substance (Coecke et al. 2006).

Unresolved scientific issues of that type are potential barriers to full validation and acceptance of some new concepts and methods for use in the regulatory context. Such issues show that although the vision conforms to the current movement from in vivo to in vitro test systems, a new set of scientific and related issues may replace interspecies extrapolation as a source of controversy. For example, using human cell lines in culture instead of laboratory animals to identify early perturbations in a cellular-response network avoids the uncertainties associated with the customary animal-to-human extrapolation. But such human-to-human methods introduce new issues and related uncertainties, such as extrapolation from isolated cells in tissue culture to intact humans and from the genetic backgrounds of the cultured cells to the genetic backgrounds of individuals or populations of interest for risk-assessment purposes.

Incorporation of emerging methods depends in part on the status of the new methods in the scientific community, which in turn depends on the reliability of new test systems in identifying compounds with known biologic activities. The generic question is "readiness" for regulatory use. Methods still under development are not necessarily barred, but until they are fully tested and documentable, questions regarding extrapolation, relevance, and possible controversy with respect to use for regulatory purposes can be expected.

Identifying and Defining Markers and Indicators of Adverse Responses

The vision calls for replacing current tests for apical end points, such as tumors and birth defects, with mechanistically based testing that identifies early markers of disease and potential risk. The new tests focus on perturbations that are expected to produce adverse responses. This aspect of the vision presents validation issues that require two kinds of documentation, one scientific and one policy-related.

As discussed above, assessment of scientific validity will require evidence, such as peer-reviewed publications and other indicators of acceptance in the scientific community. Similar documentation will be required for other new end-point categories identified as early indicators of perturbations of critical pathways that have the potential to cause toxic effects.

The policy question is an old one: What constitutes an adverse effect? The regulatory trigger for many statutes administered by EPA is an adverse effect or some variation. For example, the Safe Drinking Water Act calls for establishing contaminant concentrations at which "no known or anticipated adverse effects on the health of persons occur and which allows an adequate margin of safety." A FIFRA provision calls for preventing "unreasonable adverse effects on the environment," a phrase that includes nontarget animals as well as humans. As a result, identifying adverse effects is the objective of many current testing practices and regulations and will be critical for the use of new test methods and data.

Historically, both in legislation and in practice, testing and regulation have focused on apical end points, particularly clinically, anatomically, or histopathologically observable end points, such as tumors, birth defects, and neurologic impairments. That precedent could provide a basis of resistance to a move from traditional apical end points to perturbations of toxicity pathways. However, despite the historical emphasis, scientific and regulatory sources make clear that adverse effects embrace a wide array of end-point categories. Table 6-1 provides some definitions that are consistent with the vision's approach to toxicity testing.

In this case, establishing validity for regulatory purposes involves documenting (1) sources that justify a broad interpretation of adverse effects as a concept and (2) published papers and other materials that show the relationship between responses in toxicity pathways and disease. Case studies that link specific chemicals, mechanistic end points, and disease would be useful.

Policy and Procedural Prerequisites of Validity

Ideally, new test systems and agency guidelines that incorporate them will co-evolve. In that regard, opportunities for public participation are as important as scientific measures of validity. For the courts, in laboratories subject to government testing requirements, and in the public forum, the perceived legitimacy of new testing approaches depends also on nonscientific factors.

TABLE 6-1 Definitions of Adverse Effect

Definition	Source
"Adverse effect: A biochemical change, functional impairment, or pathologic lesion that affects the performance of the whole organism, or reduces an organism's ability to respond to an additional environmental challenge."	IRIS 2007
"Adverse effect: Change in the morphology, physiology, growth, development or life span of an organism, system or (sub) population that results in an impairment of functional capacity, an impairment of the capacity to compensate for additional stress, or an increase in susceptibility to other external influences."	Renwick et al. 2003
". . . adverse effects are changes that are undesirable because they alter valued structural or functional attributes of the entities of interest . . . . The nature and intensity of effects help distinguish adverse changes from normal . . . variability or those resulting in little or no significant change."	Sergeant 2002
"The spectrum of undesired effects of chemicals is broad. Some effects are deleterious and others are not. . . . [Regarding drugs], some side effects . . . are never desirable and are deleterious to the well-being of humans. These are referred to as the adverse, deleterious, or toxic effects of the drug."	Klaassen and Eaton 1991
"All chemicals produce their toxic effects via alterations in normal cellular biochemistry and physiology . . . . It should also be recognized that most organs have a capacity for function that exceeds that required for normal homeostasis, sometimes referred to as functional reserve capacity."	Klaassen and Eaton 1991

Establishing a Record

For any of the components of the vision, documentary evidence of scientific validity reviewed above makes up the substantive portion of the record, but evidence of public participation is also important. Current EPA practice often includes extensive discussion with scientists in universities, industry, advocacy groups, and other government agencies at public conferences and workshops. Informal or formal notice-and-comment rule-making procedures and external peer review are critical steps in the development and issuance of new testing and risk-assessment guidance (EPA 1998b, 2005).

Audience and Communication Issues

The committee's vision is the product of extensive scientific thought supported by a substantial body of scientific evidence. The scientific principles and methods involved in the implementation of the committee's vision are well known in the scientific community, a major constituency in the discussion of the scientific validity of data derived from toxicity tests for regulatory use. Scientists have long recognized the importance of effective communication of scientific results to a wide variety of stakeholders in toxicity testing, including other scientists, regulatory authorities, industry, the mass media, nongovernment organizations, and the public (NRC 1989; Leiss 2001; Krewski et al. 2006; ATSDR 2007). However, because of the transformative nature of the committee's vision for toxicity testing, communication of the scientific basis of the vision and its implications for risk assessment of environmental agents will be challenging.

Here, there is a need for clarity in communicating the essence of the committee's vision to affected parties. The nature and scientific complexity of the unfamiliar and more sophisticated methods promoted in the vision may require new communication approaches. The scientific community may be best positioned to understand the scientific basis on which the committee's vision rests but may need time to appreciate its implications fully. Acceptance of the committee's vision in the scientific community will require further elaboration of the technical details of its implementation and generation of new scientific evidence to support the move away from apical end points to perturbations of toxicity pathways. The broad participation of the scientific community in the elaboration of the committee's vision for toxicity testing is essential for its success.

Even more challenging will be the nonscientists' understanding and acceptance of the committee's vision. Regulatory authorities will need to consider how current risk-assessment practices can be adapted to make use of the types of toxicity-testing data underlying the committee's vision to arrive at human exposure guidelines for environmental agents judged, on the basis of the new test results, to have toxic potential. Law-makers will need to determine whether the regulatory statutes that form the basis of such guidelines need to be modified to reflect the greater reliance on indicators of toxicity-pathway perturbations than on overt health outcomes. For regulatory and legal experts to support the implementation of the committee's vision, it is essential that the fundamental biologic tenets underlying it be clearly articulated and reinforced by the development of the scientific data needed to support the shift away from a focus on apical outcomes to biologic perturbations of key toxicity pathways. The communication challenge will be to portray the benefits of adopting the committee's vision in scientifically valid terms without confusing the vision with over-reliance on intricate scientific detail.

Adoption of the committee's vision will require acceptance by politicians and the public alike. There will undoubtedly be a lack of support for its implementation if the scientific essence of the vision (the notion of toxicity pathways and the effects of perturbing them) is not communicated in understandable terms. Data will need to be generated to demonstrate that avoidance of such perturbations will provide a level of protection against the potential health risks posed by environmental agents at least as great as the current level. It will also be important to demonstrate that adoption of the committee's vision will permit an assessment of the potential risks associated with many more agents than is possible with current toxicity-testing practices and that this expanded coverage of the universe of environmental agents can be achieved cost-effectively.

The vision for toxicity testing in the 21st century articulated here represents a paradigm shift from the use of experimental animals and apical end points toward the use of more efficient in vitro tests and computational techniques. Implementation of the vision, which will provide much broader coverage of the universe of environmental agents that warrant our attention from a risk-assessment perspective, will require a concerted effort on the part of the scientific community. A substantial commitment of resources will be required to generate the scientific data needed to support that paradigm shift, which can be achieved only with the steadfast support of regulators, law-makers, industry, and the general public. Their support will be garnered only if the essence of the committee's vision can be communicated to all stakeholders in understandable terms.

REFERENCES

ATSDR (Agency for Toxic Substances and Disease Registry). 2007. A Primer on Health Risk Communication Principles and Practices. U.S. Department of Health and Human Services, Agency for Toxic Substances and Disease Registry, Division of Health Education, Atlanta, GA [online]. Available: http://www.atsdr.cdc.gov/risk/ riskprimer/index.html [accessed March 20, 2007].

CalEPA (California Environmental Protection Agency). 2004. Public Health Goal for Arsenic in Drinking Water. Office of Environmental Health Hazard As-

sessment, California Environmental Protection Agency. April 2004 [online].
Available: http://www.oehha.ca.gov/water/phg/pdf/asfinal.pdf [accessed
March 20, 2007].

Coecke, S., H. Ahr, B.J. Blaauboer, S. Bremer, S. Casati, J. Castell, R. Combes, R.
Corvi, C.L. Crespi, M.L. Cunningham, G. Elaut, B. Eletti, A. Freidig, A.
Gennari, J.F. Ghersi-Egea, A. Guillouzo, T. Hartung, P. Hoet, M. Ingelman-
Sundberg, S. Munn, W. Janssens, B. Ladstetter, D. Leahy, A. Long, A. Meneguz, M. Monshouwer, S. Morath, F. Nagelkerke, O. Pelkonen, J. Ponti, P.
Prieto, L. Richert, E. Sabbioni, B. Schaack, W. Steiling, E. Testai, J.A. Vericat, and A. Worth. 2006. Metabolism: A bottleneck in *in vitro* toxicological
test development. The report and recommendations of ECVM Workshop
54. ATLA 34(1):49-84.

EPA (U.S. Environmental Protection Agency). 1991. Guidelines for Developmental Toxicity Risk Assessment. EPA/600/FR-91/001. Risk Assessment Forum,
U.S. Environmental Protection Agency, Washington, DC [online]. Available: http://www.epa.gov/NCEA/raf/pdfs/devtox.pdf [accessed March 7,
2007].

EPA (U.S. Environmental Protection Agency). 1996. Guidelines for Reproductive
Toxicity Risk Assessment. EPA/630/R-96/009. Risk Assessment Forum, U.S.
Environmental Protection Agency, Washington, DC [online]. Available:
http:://www.epa.gov/ncea/raf/pdfs/repro51.pdf [accessed July 27, 2006].

EPA (U.S. Environmental Protection Agency). 1998a. Guidelines for
Neurotoxicity Risk Assessment. EPA/630/R-95/001F. Risk Assessment
Forum, U.S. Environmental Protection Agency, Washington, DC [online].
Available: http://www.epa.gov/ncea/raf/pdfs/neurotox.pdf [accessed
March 7, 2007].

EPA (U.S. Environmental Protection Agency). 1998b. Health Effects Test
Guidelines: OPPTS 870.4300 Combined Chronic Toxicity/Carcinogenicity.
EPA 712-C-98-212. Office of Prevention, Pesticides and Toxic Substances,
U.S. Environmental Protection Agency, Washington, DC [online].
Available: http://www.epa.gov/opptsfrs/publications/OPPTS_Harmon
ized/870_Health_Effects_Test_Guidelines/Series/870-4300.pdf [accessed
March 20, 2007].

EPA (U.S. Environmental Protection Agency). 2005. Guidelines for Carcinogen
Risk Assessment. EPA/630/P-03/001F. Risk Assessment Forum, U.S. Environmental Protection Agency, Washington, DC [online]. Available:
http://www.epa.gov/iris/cancer032505.pdf [accessed July 27, 2006].

EPA (U.S. Environmental Protection Agency). 2006. Pesticides: Science and
Policy. Office of Pesticides, U.S. Environmental Protection Agency [online].
Available: http://www.epa.gov/pesticides/science/index.htm [accessed
March 21, 2007].

IARC (International Agency for Research on Cancer). 2006. Cobalt in Hard Metals and Cobalt Sulfate, Gallium Arsenide, Indium Phosphide and Vanadium Pentoxide. IARC Monographs on the Evaluation of Carcinogenic Risks to Humans, Vol. 86. Lyon, France: IARC Press.

IRIS (Integrated Risk Information System). 2007. Glossary of IRIS Terms. Integrated Risk Information System, U.S. Environmental Protection Agency [online]. Available: http://www.epa.gov/iris/gloss8.htm [accessed March 20, 2007].

Klaassen, C.D., and D.L. Eaton . 1991. Principles of toxicology. Pp. 12-49 in Casarett and Doull's Toxicology: The Basic Science of Poisons, 4th Ed., M.O. Amdur, J. Doull, and C.D. Klaassen, eds. New York: Pergamon Press.

Krewski, D., L. Lemyre, M.C. Turner, J.E.C. Lee, C. Dallaire, L. Bouchard, K. Brand, and P. Mercier. 2006. Public perception of population health risks in Canada: Health hazards and sources of information. Hum. Ecol. Risk Assess. 12(4):626-644.

Leiss, W. 2001. In the Chamber of Risks: Understanding Risk Controversies. Montreal: McGill-Queen's University Press.

Lieber, M.M. 2006. Towards an understanding of the role of forces in carcinogenesis: A perspective with therapeutic implications. Riv. Biol. 99(1):131-160.

Meek, M.E., J.R. Bucher, S.M. Cohen, V. Dellarco, R.N. Hill, L.D. Lehman-McKeeman, D.G. Longfellow, T. Pastoor, J. Seed, and D. Patton. 2003. A framework for human relevance analysis of information on carcinogenic modes of action. Crit. Rev. Toxicol. 33(6):591-653.

NRC (National Research Council). 1989. Improving Risk Communication. Washington, DC: National Academy Press.

NTP (National Toxicology Program). 2005. Report on Carcinogens, 11th Ed. U.S. Department of Health and Human Services, Public Health Service, National Toxicology Program [online]. Available: http://ntpserver.niehs.nih.gov/ntp/roc/toc11.html [accessed March 20, 2007].

Renwick, A.G., S.M Barlow, I. Hertz-Picciotto, A.R. Boobis, E. Dybing, L. Edler, G. Eisenbrand, J.B. Greig, J. Kleiner, J. Lambe, D.J. Muller, M.R. Smith, A. Tritscher, S. Tuijtelaars, P.A. van den Brandt, R. Walter, and R. Kroes. 2003. Risk characterization of chemicals in food and diet. Food Chem. Toxicol. 41(9):1211-1271.

Sergeant, A. 2002. Ecological risk assessment: History and fundamentals. Pp. 369-442 in Human and Ecological Risk Assessment: Theory and Practice, D.J. Paustenbach, ed. New York: John Wiley and Sons.

Appendix

Biographic Information on the Committee on Toxicity Testing and Assessment of Environmental Agents

Daniel Krewski *(Chair)* is professor of epidemiology and community medicine and director of the McLaughlin Centre for Population Health Risk Assessment at the University of Ottawa. Previously, he served as director of the Bureau of Chemical Hazards and director of risk management at Health Canada. His research interests include epidemiology, biostatistics, risk assessment, and risk management. Dr. Krewski is a member of the National Research Council (NRC) Nuclear and Radiation Studies Board and previously served on its Committee on Health Risks of Exposure to Radon (BEIR VI) and its Committee to Assess Health Risks from Exposure to Low Levels of Ionizing Radiation (BEIR VII, Phase 2). Dr. Krewski also served on the Board on Environmental Studies and Toxicology, the Committee on Research Priorities for Airborne Particulate Matter, the Committee on Grand Challenges in Environmental Science, the Committee on Comparative Toxicity of Naturally Occurring Carcinogens, the Committee on Toxicology (COT), the COT Subcommittee on the Health Effects of Ingested Fluoride, and the Subcommittee on Pharmacokinetics in Risk Assessment of the Safe Drinking Water Committee. Dr. Krewski chaired the Committee on Acute Exposure Guideline Levels from 1998 to 2004, and the Colloquium on Scientific Advances and the Future of Toxicologic Risk Assessment held in 1997 on the 50th anniversary of the COT. Dr. Krewski received his MSc and PhD in mathematics and statistics from Carleton University and his MHA from the University of Ottawa.

Daniel Acosta, Jr. is dean of the College of Pharmacy at the University of Cincinnati. Dr. Acosta's research focuses on the development of in vitro cellular models to explore and evaluate the mechanisms by which xenobiotics damage cell types. He has worked to develop primary culture systems of liver, heart, kidney, nerve, skin, and eye cells as experimental models to study the cellular and subcellular toxicity of selected xenobiotics. He was president of the Society of Toxicology in 2000-2001 and is editor of *Toxicology In Vitro* and the *Target Organ Series on Cardiovascular Toxicology*. Dr. Acosta serves as chair of the Food and Drug Administration Scientific Advisory Board for the National Center for Toxicology Research and was a member of the Board of Scientific Councilors for the Office of Research and Development for the Environmental Protection Agency in 2001-2004. He was a member of the Scientific Advisory Committee to the director of the National Center for Environmental Health of the Centers for Disease Control and Prevention in 2001-2003. He is serving on the Scientific Advisory Committee for Alternative Toxicological Methods for the National Institute of Environmental Health Sciences and the Expert Committee on Toxicology and Biocompatibility for the US Pharmacopoeia (2000-2005). He also served on the National Research Council Howard Hughes Medical Institute Predoctoral Fellowships Panel on Neurosciences and Physiology. Dr. Acosta received his PhD in pharmacology and toxicology from the University of Kansas.

Melvin Andersen is director of the Computational Biology Division at the Hamner Institutes for Health Sciences. Previously, he held positions in toxicology research and research management in the federal government (Department of Defense and Environmental Protection Agency) and was professor of environmental health at Colorado State University. He has worked to develop biologically realistic models of the uptake, distribution, metabolism, and biologic effects of drugs and toxic chemicals and has applied these physiologically based pharmacokinetic and pharmacodynamic models to safety assessments and quantitative health risk assessments. His current research interests include developing mathematical descriptions of control of genetic circuitry in the developing and adult organism and the dose-response and risk-assessment implications of the control processes. Dr. Andersen is board-certified in industrial hygiene and in toxicology. He has served on numerous National Research Council committees, including the Committee on Toxicology, the Committee on Toxicological Effects of Mercury, the Committee on Risk Assessment Methodology, and the Subcommittee on Pharmacokinetics. He earned a PhD in biochemistry and molecular biology from Cornell University.

Henry Anderson is chief medical officer and state epidemiologist for occupational and environmental health in the Wisconsin Division of Public Health and adjunct professor of population health at the University of Wisconsin Medical School. Dr. Anderson's research interests include disease surveillance, risk assessment, childhood asthma, lead poisoning, health hazards of Great Lakes sport-fish consumption, arsenic in drinking water, bioterrorism, asbestos disease, vermiculite exposure, and occupational fatalities and injuries in youth. He is certified by the American Board of

Preventive Medicine with a subspecialty in occupational and environmental medicine and is a fellow of the American College of Epidemiology. Dr. Anderson is chair of the Board of Scientific Councilors of the National Institute for Occupational Safety and Health and has served as chair of the Environmental Health Committee of the Environmental Protection Agency Scientific Advisory Board. He served on the National Research Council Committee on a National Agenda for the Prevention of Disabilities and Committee on Enhancing Environmental Health Content in Nursing Practice. Dr. Anderson received his MD from the University of Wisconsin Medical School.

John C. Bailar III is professor emeritus in the Department of Health Studies at the University of Chicago. He is a retired commissioned officer of the U.S. Public Health Service and worked for the National Cancer Institute for 22 years. He has also held academic appointments at Harvard University and McGill University. Dr. Bailar's research interests include assessing health risks posed by chemical hazards and air pollutants and interpreting statistical evidence in medicine, with emphasis on cancer. He was editor-in-chief of the *Journal of the National Cancer Institute* for 6 years and was statistical consultant for and then member of the Editorial Board of the *New England Journal of Medicine*. Dr. Bailar is a member of the International Statistical Institute and was elected to the Institute of Medicine in 1993. He received his MD from Yale University and his PhD in statistics from American University.

Kim Boekelheide is professor in the Department of Pathology and Laboratory Medicine at Brown University. His research interests are in male reproductive biology and toxicology, particularly the potential roles of germ-cell proliferation and apoptosis and local paracrine growth factors in the regulation of spermatogenesis after toxicant-induced injury. Dr. Boekelheide serves on the National Research Council Subcommittee on

_5g

Fluoride in Drinking Water and has served on the Committee on Gender Differences in Susceptibility to Environmental Factors: A Priority Assessment. He is a past member of the Board of Scientific Counselors of the National Toxicology Program (NTP) and currently serves on the NTP Center for the Evaluation of Risks to Human Reproduction expert panel that is evaluating di-(2-ethylhexyl)phthalate. Dr. Boekelheide received his MD and PhD (in pathology) from Duke University and is board-certified in anatomic and clinical pathology.

Robert Brent is Distinguished Professor of Pediatrics, Radiology, and Pathology at the Jefferson Medical College of Thomas Jefferson University and head of the Laboratory of Clinical and Environmental Teratology at the Alfred I. duPont Hospital for Children. Dr. Brent's research focuses on the environmental and genetic causes of congenital malformations, genetic disease, and cancer, with an emphasis on reproduction and the toxicity of drugs, physical agents, and chemicals. Dr. Brent is the author or "The Vulnerability and Resiliency of the Developing Embryo, Infant, Child and Adolescent to the Effects of Environmental Chemicals, Drugs and Physical Agents as compared to Adults" for the Environmental Protection Agency and the American Academy of Pediatrics, which was published in *Pediatrics* in April 2004. He is a member of the Institute of Medicine. Dr. Brent received his MD with honors; a PhD in embryology, radiation biology, and physics; and an honorary DSc—all from the University of Rochester.

Gail Charnley is principal of HealthRisk Strategies, her consulting practice in Washington, DC. Her interests are toxicology, environmental health risk assessment, and risk-management science and policy. She was executive director of the Presidential/Congressional Commission on Risk Assessment and Risk Management, mandated by Congress to evaluate the role that risk assessment and risk management play in federal regulatory programs. Before her appointment to the commission, she served as director of the toxicology and risk-assessment program at the National Academies. She has been the project director for several National Research Council (NRC) committees, including the Committee on Risk Assessment Methodology and the Complex Mixtures Committee, and served as the chair of several U.S. Army Science Advisory Board committees that evaluated health risk assessment. Dr. Charnley serves on the NRC Committee on Improving Practices for Regulating and Managing Low-Activity Radioactive Waste. She received her PhD in toxicology from the Massachusetts Institute of Technology.

Vivian G. Cheung is associate professor in the Department of Pediatrics and Genetics at the University of Pennsylvania School of Medicine and a member of the Cell and Molecular Biology and Genomics and Computational Biology Graduate Groups. Her primary research interests include human-genome variation, DNA-damage repair, and the use of genomewide approaches to study the genetic basis of human phenotypes and traits. Her research techniques include genomic-mismatch scanning, sequence-mismatch detection, physical mapping, molecular fingerprinting, DNA microarrays, fluorescent image analysis, and developing genome databases. She earned her MD from Tufts University.

Sidney Green, Jr. is graduate professor of pharmacology at Howard University College of Medicine. Dr. Green's research interests include tissue culture, scientific and policy issues associated with alternatives, use of animals in toxicology, and mutagenic assay systems. He has served on the editorial boards of several scientific journals, and he is a fellow of the Academy of Toxicological Sciences. Dr. Green is a member of the National Research Council (NRC) Committee on Toxicology and has served on several NRC panels, including the Subcommittee on Acute Exposure Guideline

Levels, the Subcommittee on the Toxicity of Diisopropyl Methyl-phosphonate, and the Subcommittee on Iodotrifluoromethane. He received his PhD in biochemical pharmacology from Howard University.

Karl T. Kelsey is professor of cancer biology and environmental health in the Departments of Genetics and Complex Diseases and Environmental Health at the Harvard School of Public Health. Dr. Kelsey's research interests are in occupational and environmental disease, including susceptibility to disease, with emphasis on gene-environment interactions in the production of chronic disease, and the determinants of somatic gene inactivation in lung and upper airway cancers. He has been at the Harvard School of Public Health since 1987. Dr. Kelsey has served on numerous National Research Council committees, including the Committee on Copper in Drinking Water, the Committee to Review the Health Consequences of Service during the Persian Gulf War, and the Committee on the Health Effects of Mustard Gas and Lewisite. Dr. Kelsey received his MD from the University of Minnesota and an MOH from Harvard University.

Nancy I. Kerkvliet is a professor in the Department of Environmental and Molecular Toxicology at Oregon State University (OSU). Dr. Kerkvliet also serves as the associate director of the Environmental Health Sciences Center at OSU and director of the Flow Cytometry and Cell Sorting Facilities Core. Her research interests include the use of animal models to understand how chemicals alter immune function, particularly the mechanisms of action of polychlorinated dibenzo-*p*-dioxins and other aryl hydro-carbon receptor (AhR) ligands. Transgenic and gene-deletion approaches are being used, as well as genomics, to address mechanisms of AhR-mediated immunotoxicity. She is also active in public-outreach education programs in toxicology and risk communication. Dr. Kerkvliet is a member of the Institute of Medicine

Committee to Review the Health Effects in Vietnam Veterans of Exposure to Herbicides and is a past member of the National Research Council Committee on Toxicology. She has also served as a councilor for the Society of Toxicology. She earned her PhD in interdisciplinary biologic sciences and toxicology from OSU.

Abby A. Li recently joined Exponent, Inc. as a managing scientist-toxicologist in the health risk and food and chemical practices. Her fields of research include toxicology, neurotoxicology, developmental neurotoxicology, psychopharmacology, risk assessment, and pesticide regulation. Previously, Dr. Li was a senior science fellow and a global regulatory science manager at Monsanto, providing expertise in toxicology and risk assessment to address regulatory scientific issues in different world areas. For more than 10 years, she led the neurotoxicology group at Monsanto's Environmental Health Laboratory, where she conducted pharmacokinetic, toxicology, and neurotoxicology studies of industrial chemicals, agricultural products, and pharmaceuticals. Dr. Li served on the U.S. expert teams to the Organisation for Economic Cooperation and Development for the development of international test guidelines for adult and developmental neurotoxicology and as chair of neurotoxicology expert groups for industry trade organizations (the American Chemistry Council's long-range research program and the American Industrial Health Council) addressing scientific regulatory issues in neurotoxicology. Dr. Li was a member of the Environmental Protection Agency Science Advisory Board's Environmental Health Committee for 6 years, reviewing the lead rule, 1,3-butadiene risk assessment, trichloroethylene risk assessment, cancer guidelines, the IRIS database, development of acute reference exposure, methods for derivation of inhalation reference concentrations, and indoor-air toxics priority ranking. She is a member of the International Life Science Institute Agricultural Chemical Safety Assessment panel involved in redesign of safety assessment of pesticides. She received her PhD in pharmacology and physiology from the University of Chicago.

Lawrence McCray teaches at the Massachusetts Institute of Technology (MIT), where he leads a project on the use of knowledge in decision-making and participates in other research on organizational performance and behavior in risk management. Dr. McCray was a staff director and a senior manager at the National Research Council, where he led many studies on U.S. science and technology policy programs, including the study *Risk Assessment in the Federal Government: Managing the Process*, the so-called Red Book. Dr. McCray also served as head of the Environmental Protection Agency Regulatory Reform Unit and as a program director on regulatory reform in the Executive Office of the President. He earned a PhD in science and public policy from MIT and an MBA from Union College.

Otto Meyer is head of the Section of Biology, Department of Toxicology and Risk Assessment, the National Food Institute, Technical University of Denmark. The section has overall responsibility for in vivo testing in the department, including repeated dose-toxicity studies, carcinogenicity studies, reproductive-toxicity studies, and neurotoxicity studies. He is the specialized expert to the European Economic Community on classification and labeling of dangerous substances with carcinogenic, mutagenic, or teratogenic properties and national coordinator of the Test Guideline Programme (human health) of the Organisation for Economic Cooperation and Development (OECD). Concerning the latter commitment, Dr. Meyer is a member of the group preparing an OECD guidance document on reproductive toxicity and assessment. During the last 5 years, he has served as a member of the European Union Scientific Committee on Plant Protection Products (now named the Panel of Plant Health), Plant Protection and their Residues under the European Food Safety Authority. Dr. Meyer earned a DVM from the Royal Veterinary and Agricultural University in Copenhagen.

D. Reid Patterson retired in 2003 after almost 20 years of responsibility for the toxicity and safety assessment of the diverse portfolio of pharmaceutical, diagnostic, and hospital products for Abbott Laboratories; he is now a private consultant. During his tenure, he led the research efforts in toxicology, pathology, laboratory animal medicine, metabolism, pharmacokinetics, and analytic chemistry in an effort to characterize product hazards. Environmental toxicity was a greater focus during his earlier years in the petrochemical industry (Shell) and the contract laboratory business (Hazleton). Dr. Patterson is a veterinarian with residency training in laboratory animal medicine, and he received his PhD in comparative pathology from the University of Missouri. He is board-certified in laboratory animal medicine, veterinary pathology, and general toxicology, and he is a fellow of the Academy of Toxicological Sciences and the International Academy of Toxicologic Pathology.

William Pennie is research-site lead for drug safety at Pfizer's Connecticut laboratories. Dr. Pennie's research interests began with the molecular biology of the estrogen receptor, particularly differential transcriptional regulation by estrogen-receptor subtypes. More recently, his interests have included global receptor biology, improving the predictivity of investigative techniques used at early stages of product development, the technology and application of custom microarray toxicogenomics platforms, and the application of state-of-the-art molecular profiling techniques to research and investigative toxicology. He chaired the International Life Sciences Institute Health and Environmental Sciences Institute (ILSI HESI) Committee on the Application of Genomics to Mechanism-Based Risk Assessment from 2002 to 2004. Dr. Pennie received his PhD from the Beatson Institute for Cancer Research at the University of Glasgow, Scotland.

Robert A. Scala is former senior scientific adviser at Exxon Biomedical Sciences Inc. He is also an adjunct professor of toxicology at Rutgers University. He is well known for his work on the toxicity of gasoline components and chemical mixtures. He is a past president of the Society of Toxicology and the American Board of Toxicology. He has published in chronic toxicity testing and evaluation of alternative test protocols and data. Dr. Scala has served on several National Research Council committees, including the Committee on Environmental Justice: Research, Education, and Health Policy Needs, the Committee on Lead Toxicity, and the Committee on Methods for In Vivo Toxicity Testing of Complex Mixtures from the Environment. Dr. Scala earned his PhD in physiology from the University of Rochester School of Medicine and Dentistry.

Gina M. Solomon is a senior scientist at the Natural Resources Defense Council and an associate clinical professor of medicine at the University of California, San Francisco (UCSF), where she is also the associate director of the UCSF Pediatric Environmental Health Specialty Unit. Her work has included research on asthma, pesticides, and environmental and occupational threats to reproductive health and child development. Dr. Solomon serves on the Environmental Protection Agency Science Advisory Board Drinking Water Committee and previously served on the Endocrine Disruptor Screening and Testing Advisory Committee. Dr. Solomon received her MD from Yale University and underwent her postgraduate training in medicine and public health at Harvard University.

Martin Stephens is vice president of the Animal Research Issues Section of the Humane Society of the United States. Dr. Stephens serves as coordinator of the International Council for Animal Protection at the Organisation for Economic Co-operations and Development. He also serves on the Scientific Advisory Committee on Alternative Toxicological Methods for the National Toxicology Program Interagency Center for the Evaluation of Alternative Toxicological Methods and on the Scientific Advisory Panel of the Institute for In Vitro Sciences. Dr. Stephens has extensive experience in animal protection and in vitro testing sciences. He earned a PhD in biology from the University of Chicago.

James Yager is professor of toxicology in the Department of Environmental Health Sciences, director of the National Institute of Environmental Health Sciences Training Program in Environmental Health Sciences, and senior associate dean for academic affairs at the Johns Hopkins University Bloomberg School of Public Health. Dr. Yager is a member and a past president of the carcinogenesis specialty section of the Society of Toxicology. His research focuses on the role of catechol metabolites of endogenous, synthetic, and environmental estrogens and polymorphisms in genes involved in estrogen metabolism as risk factors in the development of cancer of the breast and liver. Dr. Yager earned his PhD from the University of Connecticut.

Lauren Zeise is chief of the Reproductive and Cancer Hazard Assessment Branch of the California Environmental Protection Agency. Dr. Zeise's research focuses on modeling human interindividual variability and risk. She has served on advisory boards of the U.S. Environmental Protection Agency (EPA), the World Health Organization, the Office of Technology and Assessment, and the National Institute of Environmental Health Sciences. She has also served on several National Research Council committees, including the Committee on Risk Characterization, the Committee on Comparative Toxicology of Naturally Occurring Carcinogens, the Committee on Copper in Drinking Water, and the Committee to Review EPA's Research Grants Program. Dr. Zeise is a member of the Board on Environmental Studies and Toxicology. She received her PhD from Harvard University.